The Pocket

FAT

COUNTER

SECOND EDITION

Revised and Updated

ANNETTE B. NATOW, Ph.D., R.D.
and JO-ANN HESLIN, M.A., R.D.

POCKET BOOKS

New York London Toronto Sydney Tokyo Singapore

POCKET BOOKS, a division of Simon & Schuster Inc.
1230 Avenue of the Americas, New York, NY 10020

ISBN: 0-671-00450-6

First Pocket Books printing of this revised edition May 1998

10 9 8 7 6 5 4 3 2 1

POCKET and colophon are registered trademarks of Simon & Schuster Inc.

Cover design by Tom McKeveny

Printed in the U.S.A.

THE POCKET
Fat Counter

We know we eat more fat than is good for us, and we want to do something about it—which is why we use *The Fat Counter.* Now, with *THE POCKET FAT COUNTER,* we won't ever have to wonder how much fat is in an item at the supermarket or in a restaurant. *THE POCKET FAT COUNTER* makes it deliciously easy to live a healthy, lowfat lifestyle while keeping on the move.

ANNETTE B. NATOW, Ph.D., R.D., and JO-ANN HESLIN, M.A., R.D., are the authors of twenty-one books on nutrition. Both are former faculty members of Adelphi University and the State University of New York, Downstate Medical Center. They are editors of the *Journal of Nutrition for the Elderly*, serve as editorial board members for the *Environmental Nutrition Newsletter*, and are contributors to magazines and journals.

Books by Annette B. Natow and Jo-Ann Heslin

The Antioxidant Vitamin Counter
The Calorie Counter
The Cholesterol Counter (Fourth Edition)
The Diabetes Carbohydrate and Calorie Counter
The Fast Food Nutrition Counter
The Fat Attack Plan
The Fat Counter (Fourth Edition)
The Iron Counter
Megadoses
No-Nonsense Nutrition for Kids
The Pocket Encyclopedia of Nutrition
The Pocket Fat Counter (Second Edition)
The Pocket Protein Counter
The Pregnancy Nutrition Counter
The Protein Counter
The Sodium Counter
The Supermarket Nutrition Counter (Second Edition)

Published by POCKET BOOKS

For orders other than by individual consumers, Pocket Books grants a discount on the purchase of **10 or more** copies of single titles for special markets or premium use. For further details, please write to the Vice-President of Special Markets, Pocket Books, 1633 Broadway, New York, NY 10019-6785, 8th Floor.

For information on how individual consumers can place orders, please write to Mail Order Department, Simon & Schuster Inc., 200 Old Tappan Road, Old Tappan, NJ 07675.

To our families, who support us through every project: Harry, Allen, Irene, Sarah, Meryl, Laura, Marty, George, Emily, Steven, Joseph, Kristen and Karen

Acknowledgments

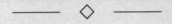

Without the tireless cooperation of Steven and Stephen, *The Pocket Fat Counter* would never have been completed. A special thanks to our editor, Jane Cavolina, and our agent, Nancy Trichter.

Our thanks also go to all the food manufacturers who graciously shared their data.

"Foods very high in fuel value, i.e., fats, and dishes containing much fat should be avoided."

Mary Swartz Rose, Ph.D.
Feeding the Family
The Macmillan Company, 1919

Sources of Data

Values in this counter have been obtained from the Composition of Foods, United States Department of Agriculture, Agricultural Handbooks: No. 8-1, Dairy and Egg Products; No. 8-2, Spices and Herbs; No. 8-3, Baby Foods; No. 8-4, Fats and Oils; No. 8-5, Poultry Products; No. 8-6, Soups, Sauces and Gravies; No. 8-7, Sausages and Luncheon Meats; No. 8-8, Breakfast Cereals; No. 8-9 Fruit and Fruit Juices; No. 8-10, Pork Products; No. 8-11, Vegetables and Vegetable Products; No. 8-12, Nut and Seed Products; No. 8-13, Beef Products; No. 8-14, Beverages; No. 8-15, Finfish and Shellfish Products; No. 8-16, Legumes and Legume Products; No. 8-17, Lamb, Veal and Game Products; No. 8-19, Snacks and Sweets; No. 8-20, Cereal Grains and Pasta; No. 8-21, Fast Foods; Supplements 1989, 1990, 1991, 1992.

Nutritive value of foods, United States Department of Agriculture, Home and Garden Bulletin No. 72.

J. Davies and J. Dickerson, *Nutrient Content of Food Portions*. Cambridge, UK: The Royal Society of Chemistry, 1991.

G. A. Leveille, M. E. Zabik, K. J. Morgan, *Nutrients in Foods*. Cambridge, MA: The Nutrition Guild, 1983.

Souci, Fachmann, Kraut, *Food Composition and Nutrition Tables*. Stuttgart: Wissenschaftliche Verlagsgesellschaft MbH, 1989.

Information from food labels, manufacturers and processors. The values are based on research conducted during 1997. Manufacturers' ingredients are subject to change, so current values may vary from those listed in the book.

INTRODUCTION

How can this book help me?

All the information you need about fat is in your pocket. The message is clear—eating less fat is better for you. Eating a lot of fat is not healthy. It causes most of the deaths in this country. Heart attacks, strokes, some cancers, diabetes, gallbladder disease, osteoarthritis and gout are some of the health problems caused or aggravated by high fat intake. And high-fat diets lead to overweight, which is a health risk by itself.

But don't I need some fat?

Yes, you do need a small amount of fat for good health, but you really can't avoid getting this small amount of fat. There is some fat—more or less—in almost all of the foods we eat.

Is it true that oils are good for me?

Foods that contain polyunsaturated and monounsaturated fats—oils, nuts, olives, fish—are better choices than foods high in saturated fats, like whole milk, cheese, butter, deli meats and regular ice cream. Most saturated fats raise blood cholesterol levels, increasing the risk for heart attack. Research suggests that too much polyunsaturated fat may cause gallbladder disease and depress the immune system. While monounsaturated fat seems to be a healthier choice, it does contain the same amount of calories as any other fat, so it's not good to eat too much.

Once you have eaten a small amount of fat, there really is no benefit in having more. The best advice is to eat less fat. *The Pocket Fat Counter* will help you do this when you are on the move throughout your busy days. With *The Pocket Fat Counter* in your pocket or bag you'll never have to wonder how much fat is in an item you are choosing in a restaurant or supermarket. You can still enjoy having your favorites and trying new dishes, if you follow some simple guidelines that won't take the fun out of eating.

One way to recognize foods high in fat is to look at the ingredient list. Lard, suet, chicken fat, butter, cocoa butter, cream, cheese, whole milk, diglycerides, fat, hydrogenated fat, hydrogenated oil, margarine, monoglycerides, oil, partially hydrogenated fat, partially hydrogenated oil, shortening, vegetable fat and vegetable oil are all fats.

Terms used on labels can be confusing. *Fat free* on a label means that there is less than one-half gram of fat in a serving of that food. This is a very small amount of fat, but the serving size may be fairly small as well, much less than the amount you usually eat. Also "fat free" does not equal "calorie free." Eating less fat helps keep you healthy, but you can't ignore the calories in foods if you want to maintain or get to your best weight. Foods labeled *fat free, lowfat* or *light* may still contain lots of calories.

TIPS TO LOWER FAT INTAKE WHEN EATING OUT

Have Food Naked

• Enjoy bread and rolls, but have them naked. Ask the waiter to take the butter away.

• Enjoy salad naked, minus regular dressing. Ask for lowfat or fat-free dressing, flavored vinegar or a squeeze of lemon.

• Enjoy a single burger, hold the sauce, cheese and bacon. Dress it with lettuce, tomatoes, onions, pickles, and ketchup or barbecue sauce.

• Enjoy pizza, but hold the extra cheese, sausage and pepperoni. Ask for peppers, onions or mushrooms instead.

- Enjoy baked or broiled fish. Ask for sauce on the side and some extra lemon wedges.
- Enjoy grilled or roast chicken. Remove the skin and hold the creamy dressing; use barbecue sauce, salsa or ketchup instead.
- Enjoy pasta with marinara, fresh tomato sauce or topped with vegetables. Skip the creamy white and meat sauces.
- Enjoy clear noodle or vegetable soup. Steer clear of cream soups and bisque.
- Enjoy pancakes with syrup, but hold the butter.
- Enjoy regular-size muffins, and skip the butter.
- Enjoy your favorite pie. Eat the filling, leave the crust.
- Enjoy coffee or tea. Ask for milk instead of cream.

Paper napkins have lots of uses. Place a muffin or other pastry on one. If it leaves a grease ring, you'll know the pastry has lots of fat. You can also use a paper napkin to blot off the oil that often pools on top of pizza. Fries will give up some of their fat when placed on a paper napkin.

TIPS FOR BUYING LOWER-FAT FOODS

- Choose fat-free, nonfat, lowfat or reduced-fat milk and lowfat or nonfat yogurt.
- Choose skim-milk, reduced-fat or fat-free cheese. Those labeled part skim milk still may be fairly high in fat.
- Choose lean meats trimmed of all visible fat and ground meat labeled "lean" or "extra lean."
- Choose poultry without skin and ground poultry made with all white

meat. Don't assume that sausage or deli meat made with poultry is low in fat; check the label. The same is true of meat substitutes, which may not be low in fat.

• Choose lean fish like cod, scrod, haddock and halibut. When using fatty fish like salmon, bluefish or mackerel, remove the skin and all visible fat.

• Choose fruit butters, fruit preserves, jelly and honey to use as a spread instead of butter or margarine.

• Choose cooking sprays and butter flavor sprinkles to replace or reduce some of the oil and butter you use.

• Choose bagels, English muffins and raisin bread for lowfat snacks instead of regular sweet rolls and doughnuts.

• Choose dried fruits—raisins, apples, prunes, peaches, apricots—for fat-free snacks.

• Choose baked chips—potato and corn—instead of the usual fried versions.

• Choose pretzels, rice cakes or air-popped popcorn for a very low fat snack.

• Choose hard candy, marshmallows, gum drops, candy corn, licorice or presweetened ready-to-eat cereals for a lowfat sweet treat.

TOP TEN FAT-FREE FAVORITES

Angelfood cake   Rice cakes
Jelly beans   Italian ices
Apple butter   Espresso
Romaine   Strawberries
Fruit nectar   Champagne

USING YOUR POCKET FAT COUNTER

This books lists the saturated fat, total fat and calorie content of over 2,000 foods. With *The Pocket Fat Counter* in your pocket, it's easy to choose lowfat foods. Because of this book's size, you may not always find your favorite brands listed. You will find enough—a few typical brand names and nonbranded samples—to make a good estimate of the fat content of your favorite brand.

All foods are listed alphabetically, A to Z. The nonbranded (generic) are first, followed by brand-name foods. Many meat and fish entries are given in 3-ounce portions. They are equal in size to a deck of cards or a tape cassette.

When you need a bigger reference—one with counts for over 21,000 foods—go to *The Fat Counter*, now in its fourth edition. We've included two blank pages so you can add counts for other foods from *The Fat Counter* into *The Pocket Fat Counter*.

DEFINITIONS

as prep (as prepared): refers to food that has been prepared according to package directions

lean and fat: describes meat with some fat on its edges that is not cut away before cooking or poultry prepared with skin and fat as purchased

lean only: lean portion, trimmed of all visible fat

tr (trace): value used when a food contains less than one calorie or less than one gram of saturated fat or total fat.

ABBREVIATIONS

avg = average
diam = diameter
fl = fluid
frzn = frozen
g = gram
in = inch
lb = pound
lg = large
med = medium
mg = milligram
oz = ounce
pkg = package
prep = prepared
pt = pint
qt = quart
reg = regular
serv = serving
sm = small
sq = square
tbsp = tablespoon
tr = trace
tsp = teaspoon
w/ = with
w/o = without
< = less than

EQUIVALENT MEASURES

DRY

3 teaspoons	= 1 tablespoon
4 tablespoons	= 1/4 cup
8 tablespoons	= 1/2 cup
12 tablespoons	= 3/4 cup
16 tablespoons	= 1 cup

1000 milligrams	= 1 gram
28 grams	= 1 ounce
4 ounces	= 1/4 pound
8 ounces	= 1/2 pound
12 ounces	= 3/4 pound
16 ounces	= 1 pound

LIQUID

2 tablespoons	= 1 ounce
2 ounces	= 1/4 cup
4 ounces	= 1/2 cup
6 ounces	= 3/4 cup
8 ounces	= 1 cup
2 cups	= 1 pint
4 cups	= 1 quart

NOTES

ALL FAT AND SATURATED FAT VALUES OF FOODS ARE GIVEN IN GRAMS (G).

A DASH (—) INDICATES DATA NOT AVAILABLE.

Discrepancies in figures are due to rounding, product reformulation and reevaluation.

If you are an average-weight, moderately active adult and want a quick benchmark for total fat grams each day simply divide your weight in half.

For example: If you weigh 120 pounds, you should have no more than 60 grams of fat a day (120 ÷ 2).

EXTRA FAT COUNTS

FOOD	PORTION	CALS.	SAT. FAT	TOTAL FAT

EXTRA FAT COUNTS

FOOD	PORTION	CALS.	SAT. FAT	TOTAL FAT

FOOD	PORTION	CALS.	SAT. FAT	TOTAL FAT
ALFALFA				
sprouts	1 tbsp	1	0	tr
ALMONDS				
oil roasted	1 oz	174	2	16
ANCHOVY				
canned in oil	5	42	tr	2
APPLE				
dried rings	10	155	tr	tr
fresh	1	81	tr	tr
Tastee Caramel Apple	1 (3 oz)	160	2	5
APPLE JUICE				
frzn as prep	1 cup	111	tr	tr
After The Fall Organic	1 bottle (10 oz)	110	0	0
Tropicana Season's Best	1 container (8 fl oz)	110	0	0
APPLESAUCE				
sweetened	½ cup	97	tr	tr
Mott's Fruit Snacks Cinnamon	4 oz	90	0	0
APRICOT JUICE				
nectar	1 cup	141	tr	tr
APRICOTS				
canned juice pack w/ skin	3 halves	40	tr	tr
dried halves	10	83	tr	tr
fresh	3	51	tr	tr
ARTICHOKE				
fresh cooked	1 med (4 oz)	60	tr	tr
Birds Eye Hearts Deluxe	½ cup	30	0	0
Progresso Hearts Marinated	⅓ cup (3 oz)	160	2	14
ARUGULA (ROCKET)				
raw	½ cup	2	0	tr
ASPARAGUS				
canned spears	½ cup	24	tr	1
fresh cooked	4 spears	14	tr	tr
Birds Eye Cut	½ cup	23	0	0
AVOCADO				
fresh	1	324	5	31
BACON				
cooked	3 strips	109	3	9

FOOD	PORTION	CALS.	SAT. FAT	TOTAL FAT
Armour Lower Salt cooked	1 strip	38	—	3
Hormel Bacon Bits	1 tsp (7 g)	30	1	2
BACON SUBSTITUTES				
Bac-Os Pieces	2 tsp (5 g)	25	0	1
Morningstar Farms Breakfast Strips	3 (25 g)	80	0	6
BAGEL				
cinnamon raisin	1 (3½ in)	194	tr	1
plain	1 (3½ in)	195	tr	1
BAMBOO SHOOTS				
Empress Sliced	2 oz	14	0	0
BANANA				
banana chips	1 oz	147	8	10
Chiquita Fresh	1 (3½ oz)	110	0	0
BARBECUE SAUCE				
Healthy Choice Original	2 tbsp (1.1 oz)	25	0	0
BASS				
striped baked	3 oz	105	1	3
BEANS				
baked beans vegetarian	½ cup	118	tr	1
B&M 99% Fat Free Baked Beans	½ cup (4.6 oz)	160	0	1
Green Giant Three Bean Salad	½ cup	70	0	tr
Old El Paso Refried Fat Free	½ cup (4.4 oz)	110	0	0
Van Camp's Baked Beans Fat Free	½ cup (4.6 oz)	130	0	0
BEEF				
bottom round lean & fat trim ¼ in Choice braised	3 oz	241	6	15
brisket whole lean & fat trim ¼ in braised	3 oz	327	11	27
corned beef brisket cooked	3 oz	213	5	16
eye of round lean & fat trim ¼ in Choice roasted	3 oz	205	5	12
flank lean & fat trim 0 in broiled	3 oz	192	5	11
ground extra lean broiled medium	3 oz	217	5	14
ground lean broiled medium	3 oz	231	6	16
porterhouse steak lean & fat trim ¼ in Choice broiled	3 oz	260	8	19
roast beef medium	2 oz	70	1	2

FOOD	PORTION	CALS.	SAT. FAT	TOTAL FAT
short ribs lean & fat Choice braised	3 oz	400	15	36
t-bone steak lean & fat trim ¼ in Choice broiled	3 oz	253	7	18
tenderloin lean & fat trim ¼ in Choice broiled	3 oz	259	7	19
top round lean & fat trim ¼ in Choice braised	3 oz	221	4	11
Hormel Dried Sliced	10 slices (1 oz)	50	1	2
BEEF DISHES				
bubble & squeak	5 oz	186	—	13
irish stew	1 cup (7 oz)	280	9	16
roast beef sandwich plain	1	346	4	14
roast beef sandwich w/ cheese	1	402	9	18
roast beef submarine sandwich w/ tomato lettuce & mayonnaise	1	411	7	13
samosa	2 (4 oz)	652	—	62
shepherds pie	6 oz	196	—	10
steak sandwich w/ tomato lettuce salt & mayonnaise	1	459	4	14
stew w/ vegetables	1 cup	220	4	11
swiss steak	4.6 oz	214	3	9
Casbah Gyro as prep	1 patty (2 oz)	145	2	5
Dinty Moore Beef Stew	1 can (7.5 oz)	190	4	10
Hot Pocket Stuffed Sandwich Barbecue	1 (4.5 oz)	340	5	12
Lean Pockets Stuffed Sandwich Beef & Broccoli	1 (4.5 oz)	250	3	7
Weight Watchers Reuben Pocket Sandwich	1 (5 oz)	250	2	6
BEER AND ALE				
alcohol free beer	7 fl oz	50	0	tr
ale brown	10 oz	77	0	0
ale pale	10 oz	88	0	0
beer light	12 oz can	100	0	0
beer regular	12 oz can	146	0	0
stout	10 oz	102	0	0
BEETS				
greens cooked	½ cup	20	tr	tr

FOOD	PORTION	CALS.	SAT. FAT	TOTAL FAT
sliced cooked	½ cup (3 oz)	38	tr	tr
Del Monte Pickled Crinkle Style Sliced	½ cup (4.5 oz)	80	0	0
BISCUIT				
plain	1 (2 oz)	212	3	10
w/ egg	1	315	6	20
w/ egg & bacon	1	457	10	31
w/ egg & sausage	1	582	15	39
BLACKEYE PEAS				
Allen Blackeye Peas	½ cup (4.5 oz)	110	1	1
BLINTZE				
Golden Cheese	1 (2.25 oz)	80	1	2
BLUEBERRIES				
fresh	1 cup	82	0	1
BOK CHOY				
Dole Shredded	½ cup	5	0	tr
BRAN				
oat cooked	½ cup	44	tr	tr
Kretschmer Toasted Wheat Bran	⅓ cup	57	tr	2
BRAZIL NUTS				
dried	1 oz	186	5	19
BREAD				
banana	1 slice (2 oz)	195	1	6
chapatis as prep w/ fat	1 (2.5 oz)	230	—	9
corn bread	2 in x 2 in (1.4 oz)	107	1	2
focaccia onion	1 piece (4.6 oz)	282	1	10
focaccia rosemary	1 piece (3.5 oz)	251	1	7
focaccia tomato olive	1 piece (4.7 oz)	270	1	8
french	1 slice (1 oz)	78	tr	1
irish soda bread	1 slice (2 oz)	174	1	3
italian	1 slice (1 oz)	81	tr	1
papadums fried	2 (1.5 oz)	81	—	4
paratha	1 (4.4 oz)	403	—	18
pita	1 reg (2 oz)	165	tr	1
pita	1 sm (1 oz)	78	tr	tr
raisin	1 slice	71	tr	1
rye	1 slice	83	tr	1
rye reduced calorie	1 slice	47	tr	1

FOOD	PORTION	CALS.	SAT. FAT	TOTAL FAT
seven grain	1 slice	65	tr	1
sourdough	1 slice (1 oz)	78	tr	1
white	1 slice	67	tr	1
white reduced calorie	1 slice	48	tr	1
whole wheat	1 slice	70	tr	1
Arnold Pumpernickel	l slice (1.1 oz)	70	0	1
Damascus Bakeries Mountain Shepard Lahvash	⅓ loaf (2 oz)	135	0	0
Freihofer's Country Potato	1 slice (1.3 oz)	100	0	1
Kontos Nan Onion	1 loaf (2.8 oz)	240	1	7
Tree Of Life 100% Spelt	1 slice (1.8 oz)	130	1	3
BREADSTICKS				
Keebler Sesame	2	30	tr	1
Stella D'Oro Deli Original Fat Free	5	60	0	0
Stella D'Oro Regular	1	40	—	1
BREAKFAST BAR				
Carnation Chewy Chocolate Chip	1 (1.26 oz)	150	3	6
Glenny's Sunrise Bee Pollen	1 (1.5 oz)	190	—	8
Nutri-Grain Raspberry	1 (1.3 oz)	140	1	3
BREAKFAST DRINKS				
Carnation Instant Breakfast Creamy Milk Chocolate	8 fl oz	220	2	3
Pillsbury Instant Breakfast Strawberry as prep w/ milk	1 serv	290	—	9
Pillsbury Instant Breakfast Vanilla as prep w/ whole milk	1 serv	300	—	9
BROCCOFLOWER				
Dole Green fresh	⅕ head	35	0	0
BROCCOLI				
chopped cooked	½ cup	22	tr	tr
Birds Eye Florets Deluxe	½ cup	25	0	0
Dole Spear	1 med	40	0	1
Green Giant In Cheese Sauce	½ cup	60	tr	2
BROWNIE				
plain	1 (0.8 oz)	112	2	7
w/nuts	1 (0.8 oz)	95	1	6
Hostess Brownie Bites Walnut	5 (2 oz)	270	4	15
Sweet Rewards Double Fudge	1 (1.1 oz)	110	0	0

FOOD	PORTION	CALS.	SAT. FAT	TOTAL FAT
Tastykake Brownie	1 (85 g)	340	3	14
Weight Watchers Brownie A La Mode	1 (6.42 oz)	190	1	4
BUCKWHEAT				
groats roasted cooked	½ cup	91	tr	tr
Wolff's Kasha Medium cooked	¼ cup (1.6 oz)	170	0	2
BULGUR				
cooked	½ cup	76	tr	tr
BUTTER				
stick	1 pat	36	3	4
whipped	1 pat	27	2	3
Land O'Lakes Light Stick	1 tbsp	50	4	6
BUTTER BEANS				
Allen Baby	½ cup (4.5 oz)	120	1	1
BUTTER BLENDS				
Country Morning Blend Light Tub	1 tbsp (0.5 oz)	50	3	6
Touch Of Butter Tub	1 tbsp (0.5 oz)	60	2	7
BUTTER SUBSTITUTES				
Butter Buds Sprinkles	1 tsp (2 g)	5	0	0
BUTTERFISH				
baked	3 oz	159	—	9
BUTTERSCOTCH				
Nestle Morsels Butterscotch	1 tbsp	80	4	4
CABBAGE				
chinese pak-choi shredded cooked	½ cup	10	tr	tr
coleslaw	½ cup	42	tr	2
green raw shredded	½ cup (1.2 oz)	9	tr	tr
green shredded cooked	½ cup (2.6 oz)	17	tr	tr
health salad	3.5 oz	150	1	9
red raw shredded	½ cup	10	tr	tr
stuffed cabbage	1 (6 oz)	373	12	22
sweet & sour red cabbage	4 oz	61	—	3
Dole Napa shredded	½ cup	6	0	tr
Fresh Express Cole Slaw w/o dressing	1½ cups (3 oz)	25	0	0
CAKE				
angelfood	1/12 cake (1.9 oz)	142	tr	tr

FOOD	PORTION	CALS.	SAT. FAT	TOTAL FAT
apple crisp	½ cup (5 oz)	230	1	5
baklava	1 oz	126	4	9
boston cream pie	⅛ cake (3.2 oz)	232	2	8
carrot w/ cream cheese icing	1/12 cake (3.9 oz)	484	5	29
cheesecake	1/12 cake (4.5 oz)	456	9	18
chocolate w/ chocolate frosting	⅛ cake (2.2 oz)	235	3	11
cream puff w/ custard filling	1 (4.6 oz)	336	5	20
eclair	1	205	—	10
fruitcake	1/36 cake (2.9 oz)	302	1	10
panettone dal forno	⅑ cake (1.9 oz)	212	4	8
pineapple upside down	⅑ cake (4 oz)	367	3	14
sponge	1/12 cake (2.2 oz)	140	1	2
strudel	1 piece (4.1 oz)	272	4	8
tiramisu	1 piece (5.1 oz)	409	15	30
Baby Watson Cheesecake	1 slice (3.8 oz)	390	18	30
Baby Watson Cheesecake Light	1/16 cake (3.9 oz)	280	9	16
Drake's Devil Dog	1 (1.5 oz)	160	—	6
Drake's Ring Ding	1 (1.5 oz)	180	—	10
Drake's Yankee Doodle	1 (1 oz)	100	—	4
Dutch Mill Dessert Shells Chocolate Covered	1 (0.5 oz)	80	2	5
Entenmann's Cinnamon Buns	1 (2.1 oz)	230	—	10
Entenmann's Coffee Cake Cheese Filled Crumb	1 serv (1.4 oz)	130	—	6
Freihofer's Coffee Cake Cinnamon Pecan	⅛ cake (2 oz)	220	2	9
Greenfield Blondie Apple Spice	1 (1.4 oz)	120	0	0
Hostess Crumb Cake Light	1 (1.8 oz)	150	0	1
Hostess Cup Cakes Chocolate	1 (1.6 oz)	170	3	5
Hostess Cup Cakes Chocolate Light	1 (1.4 oz)	120	0	2
Hostess Ding Dongs	1 (1.3 oz)	160	6	9
Hostess Ho Ho's	1 (1 oz)	130	4	6
Hostess Twinkies	1 (1.4 oz)	140	2	4
Hostess Twinkies Lights	1 (1.4 oz)	120	0	2
Kellogg's Pop-Tarts Brown Sugar Cinnamon	1 (1.8 oz)	220	1	9

FOOD	PORTION	CALS.	SAT. FAT	TOTAL FAT
Kellogg's Pop-Tarts Frosted Strawberry	1 (1.8 oz)	200	2	5
Kellogg's Rice Krispies Treats	1 (0.8 oz)	90	0	2
Little Debbie Coconut Rounds	1 pkg (1.2 oz)	140	3	7
Little Debbie Devil Cremes	1 pkg (1.6 oz)	190	2	8
Little Debbie Jelly Rolls	1 pkg (2.1 oz)	230	2	7
Little Debbie Swiss Rolls	1 pkg (2.1 oz)	250	3	12
Pepperidge Farm Toaster Tart Apple Cinnamon	1	170	2	7
Sinbad Baklava	1 piece (2 oz)	337	4	20
Tastykake Chocolate Cream Filled Cupcake	1 (34 g)	130	1	5
Toast-R-Cakes Corn	1	120	—	4
Toastettes Frosted Cherry	1 (1.7 oz)	190	2	5
Weight Watchers Coffee Cake Cinnamon Streusel	1 (2.25 oz)	190	1	2
Well-Bred Loaf Banana Bread	1 slice (3.5 oz)	330	5	11
Well-Bred Loaf Marble Poundcake	1 slice (4.3 oz)	530	11	18
Well-Bred Loaf Raisin Poundcake	1 slice (4.3 oz)	460	9	15

CALZONE

cheese	1 (12 oz)	1020	24	54

CANADIAN BACON

Jones Slices	1	30	—	1

CANDY

candy corn	1 oz	105	0	0
carob bar	1 (3.1 oz)	453	7	28
fudge chocolate	1 piece (0.6 oz)	65	1	1
marzipan	3½ oz	497	—	25
pretzels chocolate covered	1 (0.4 oz)	50	1	2
truffles	1 piece (0.4 oz)	59	3	4
3 Musketeers Bar	2 fun size (1.2 oz)	140	3	4
5th Avenue Bar	1 (2.1 oz)	290	—	13
After Eight Dark Chocolate Wafer Thin Mints	1	35	—	1
Almond Joy Bar	1 (1.76 oz)	250	—	14
Baby Ruth Bar	1 (2.1 oz)	280	7	12
Breath Savers Sugar Free Spearmint	1 piece (2 g)	10	0	0

FOOD	PORTION	CALS.	SAT. FAT	TOTAL FAT
Brock Butterscotch Discs	3 pieces (0.6 oz)	70	0	0
Brock Gummy Bears	5 pieces (1.4 oz)	130	0	0
Brock Jelly Beans	12 pieces (1.4 oz)	140	0	0
Brock Sour Balls	3 pieces (0.6 oz)	70	0	0
Butterfinger Bar	1 (2.1 oz)	280	6	11
Cellas Chocolate Covered Cherries				
Milk Chocolate	2 pieces (1 oz)	110	3	4
Certs Breath Mints	1 piece (1.67 g)	6	0	0
Charms Blow Pop	1 (0.7 oz)	80	0	0
Chuckles Candy	4 pieces (1.4 oz)	140	0	0
Chunky Bar	1 (1.4 oz)	200	6	11
Dove Milk Chocolate Miniatures	7 (1.5 oz)	230	8	13
Estee Gum Drops Assorted Fruit				
Sugar Free	23 (1.4 oz)	140	0	0
Ferrero Rocher Candy	2 pieces (0.9 oz)	150	3	10
Godiva Bouchee Au Chocolat	1 piece (1.5 oz)	210	6	11
Goldenberg's Peanut Chews	3 pieces (1.3 oz)	180	2	9
Goobers Peanuts	1 pkg (1.38 oz)	210	5	13
Good & Plenty Snacksize	3 boxes (1.5 oz)	140	0	0
Heath Bar	1 (1.4 oz)	210	7	13
Hershey Bar	1 (1.55 oz)	240	—	14
Hershey Bar With Almonds	1 (1.45 oz)	230	—	14
Hershey Kisses	9 pieces (1.46 oz)	220	—	13
Jolly Rancher Candies	3 pieces (0.6 oz)	60	0	0
Joyva Halvah	1.5 oz	240	3	16
Junior Mints Candies	1 pkg (1.6 oz)	190	3	4
Kit Kat Bar	1 (1.625 oz)	250	—	13
Kraft Caramels	5 (1.4 oz)	170	1	3
Lifesavers Gummi Savers Five				
Flavor	1 pkg (1.8 oz)	160	0	0
Lifesavers Roll Five Flavor	2 pieces (5 g)	20	0	0
M&M's Peanut	1 pkg (1.7 oz)	250	5	13
M&M's Plain	1 pkg (1.7 oz)	230	10	10
Milk Duds Pieces	1 box (1.8 oz)	230	6	8
Milky Way Bar	2 fun size (1.4 oz)	180	4	7
Mounds Bar	1 (1.9 oz)	260	—	14
Mr. Goodbar Candy	1 (1.75 oz)	290	—	19

FOOD	PORTION	CALS.	SAT. FAT	TOTAL FAT
Nestle Turtles Pecan Caramel Candy	2 pieces (1.2 oz)	160	3	9
Newman's Own Organics Espresso Sweet Dark Chocolate	1 bar (1.2 oz)	190	7	12
Pearson Licorice	2 pieces (0.5 oz)	60	2	2
Pez Candy	1 roll (0.3 oz)	30	0	0
Raisinets Raisins	1 pkg (1.58 oz)	200	4	8
Reese's Peanut Butter Cups	1 (1.8 oz)	280	—	17
Reese's Pieces	1.85 oz	260	—	11
Russell Stover Assorted Creams	3 pieces (1.4 oz)	180	4	7
Skittles Original	1 pkg (2.8 oz)	250	1	3
Snickers Miniatures	4 (1.3 oz)	170	3	8
Sno-Caps Candies	1 pkg (2.3 oz)	300	8	13
Starburst Original Fruits	8 pieces (1.4 oz)	160	1	3
Sweet Escapes Triple Chocolate Wafer Bars	1 (0.7 oz)	80	2	3
Tootsie Roll Candy	1 (1 oz)	110	0	2
Tootsie Roll Pop	1 (0.6 oz)	60	0	0
Twix Caramel	1 fun size (0.5 oz)	80	2	4
Twizzlers Candy	4 pieces (1.4 oz)	130	—	1
Velamints Peppermint	1 piece (1.7 g)	5	0	0
Very Special Chocolate Bottles Liquor Filled	3 pieces (1 oz)	150	4	6
Whitman's Assorted	3 pieces (1.4 oz)	190	5	8
Whitman's Pecan Roll	1 bar (2 oz)	300	3	20
Whoppers Candy	1 pkg (1.8 oz)	230	8	10
York Peppermint Patty	1 snack size (0.5 oz)	57	1	1
CANTALOUPE				
fresh cubed	1 cup	57	0	tr
CAPERS				
Progresso Capers (drained)	1 tsp (5 g)	0	0	0
CAROB				
carob mix	3 tsp	45	0	0
CARROT JUICE				
Hain Juice	6 fl oz	80	0	0
CARROTS				
fresh baby raw	1 (½ oz)	6	tr	tr
raw shredded	½ cup	24	tr	tr

FOOD	PORTION	CALS.	SAT. FAT	TOTAL FAT
Allen Sliced	½ cup (4.5 oz)	35	0	1
CASABA				
fresh	¹⁄₁₀	43	0	tr
CASHEWS				
dry roasted salted	1 oz	163	3	13
Fisher Honey Roasted Halves	1 oz	150	3	13
CATFISH				
breaded & fried	3 oz	194	3	11
CAULIFLOWER				
flowerets raw	3 (2 oz)	14	tr	tr
fresh cooked	½ cup (2.2 oz)	14	tr	tr
Birds Eye With Cheese Sauce	½ pkg	90	2	5
Vlasic Hot & Spicy	1 oz	4	0	0
CAVIAR				
black	1 tbsp	40	—	3
red	1 tbsp	40	—	3
CELERIAC				
fresh cooked	3½ oz	25	0	tr
CELERY				
raw	1 stalk (1.3 oz)	6	tr	tr
CEREAL				
Arrowhead 4 Grain + Flax	¼ cup (1.6 oz)	150	0	2
Arrowhead Puffed Corn	1 cup (0.8 oz)	80	0	0
Cap'n Crunch Original	¾ cup	113	1	2
Chex Corn	1¼ cup (1 oz)	110	0	0
General Mills Cheerios	1¼ cup (1 oz)	110	0	2
General Mills Cheerios Honey Nut	¾ cup (1 oz)	110	0	1
General Mills Cinnamon Toast Crunch	¾ cup (1 oz)	120	—	3
General Mills Cocoa Puffs	1 cup (1 oz)	110	—	1
General Mills Golden Grahams	¾ cup (1 oz)	110	—	1
General Mills Total	1 cup (1 oz)	100	—	1
General Mills Wheaties	1 cup (1 oz)	100	—	1
Good Shepherd Spelt	1 oz	90	—	tr
Good Shepherd Spelt Flakes	1 oz	100	—	6
H-O Farina Instant	1 pkg	110	0	0
H-O Oatmeal Instant Maple Brown Sugar	1 pkg	160	0	2

FOOD	PORTION	CALS.	SAT. FAT	TOTAL FAT
Health Valley Fiber 7 Flakes With Raisins 100% Organic	½ cup (1 oz)	90	—	tr
Health Valley Oat Bran Natural Raisins & Spice	¼ cup	100	—	tr
Heartland Raisin	1 oz	130	—	4
Kashi Cereal	2 oz	177	—	1
Kashi Puffed	¾ oz	74	—	1
Kellogg's All-Bran	½ cup (1 oz)	80	0	1
Kellogg's Complete Bran Flakes	¾ cup (1 oz)	100	0	1
Kellogg's Corn Flakes	1 cup (1 oz)	110	0	0
Kellogg's Froot Loops	1 cup (1 oz)	120	1	1
Kellogg's Frosted Flakes	¾ cup (1 oz)	120	0	0
Kellogg's Product 19	1 cup (1 oz)	110	0	0
Kellogg's Raisin Bran	1 cup (1.9 oz)	170	0	1
Kellogg's Rice Krispies	1¼ cup (1 oz)	110	0	0
Kellogg's Special K	1 cup (1 oz)	110	0	0
Maypo Vermont Style	1 oz	105	tr	1
McCann's Irish Oatmeal	1 oz	110	—	2
Nabisco Cream Of Wheat Quick as prep	1 cup	120	—	0
Nabisco Shredded Wheat Spoon Size	⅔ cup (1 oz)	90	0	1
Post Fruit & Fibre Dates Raisins Walnuts With Oat Clusters	⅔ cup	120	—	2
Post Grape-Nuts	¼ cup (1 oz)	105	0	0
Pritikin Multigrain	1 pkg	160	0	2
Quaker Instant Grits White Hominy	1 pkg	79	tr	tr
Quaker Oats Old Fashion	½ cup	150	1	3
Quaker Oats Quick	½ cup	150	1	3
Quaker Puffed Rice	1 cup	54	—	tr
Quaker Puffed Wheat	1 cup	50	0	tr
Ralston Cocoa Crispy Rice	1 cup (1.8 oz)	200	0	1
Roman Meal Original	1 oz	83	tr	1
Uncle Roy's Muesli Swiss Style	½ cup (1.6 oz)	170	1	5
Weetabix Cereal	2 (1.3 oz)	142	—	1
Wheatena Cereal	⅓ cup (1.4 oz)	150	0	1

CEREAL BARS

FOOD	PORTION	CALS.	SAT. FAT	TOTAL FAT
Cap'n Crunch Bar	1 (0.8 oz)	90	1	2

FOOD	PORTION	CALS.	SAT. FAT	TOTAL FAT
Rice Krispies Chocolate Chip	1 (1 oz)	120	2	4
CHAMPAGNE				
Andre Cold Duck	1 fl oz	25	0	0
Tott's Brut	1 fl oz	20	0	0
CHAYOTE				
fresh cooked	1 cup	38	0	1
CHEESE DISHES				
cheese omelette	1 (6.8 oz)	519	—	44
macaroni & cheese	1 cup	320	—	19
CHEESE NATURAL				
bel paese	3½ oz	391	—	30
cacio di roma sheep's milk cheese	1 oz	130	6	10
emmentaler	3½ oz	403	—	30
gjetost	1 oz	132	5	8
goat semisoft	1 oz	103	6	8
limburger	1 oz	93	5	8
port du salut	1 oz	100	5	8
queso anego	1 oz	106	5	9
queso asadero	1 oz	101	5	8
queso chichuahua	1 oz	106	5	8
roquefort	1 oz	105	5	9
whey cheese	1 oz	124	5	8
yogurt cheese	1 oz	20	0	0
Alpine Lace Cheddar Reduced Fat	1 piece (1 oz)	80	3	5
Bongrain Chavrie	2 tbsp (0.8 oz)	40	2	3
Bongrain Montrachet	1 oz	70	4	6
Bresse Brie Light	1 oz	70	3	4
Brier Run Quark	1 oz	34	—	3
Cabot Cheddar	1 oz	110	6	9
Cracker Barrel Cheddar Sharp Reduced Fat	1 oz	80	3	5
Di Giorno Parmesan	2 tsp (5 g)	20	1	1
Di Giorno Romano Grated	2 tsp (5 g)	25	1	2
Friendship Farmer	2 tbsp (1 oz)	50	2	3
Friendship Hoop	2 tbsp (1 oz)	20	0	0
Frigo Mozzarella Part Skim	1 oz	80	3	5
Healthy Choice Mozzarella Shreds	¼ cup (1 oz)	45	0	0
Heluva Good Cheese Muenster	1 oz	100	6	8

FOOD	PORTION	CALS.	SAT. FAT	TOTAL FAT
Hollow Road Farms Sheep's Milk	1 oz	45	—	3
Kraft Blue	1 oz	100	6	8
Kraft Cheddar Fat Free Shredded	¼ cup (1 oz)	45	0	0
Kraft Gouda	1 oz	110	6	9
Kraft Provolone Smoke Flavor	1 oz	100	5	7
Land O'Lakes Chedarella	1 oz	100	5	8
Land O'Lakes Swiss Light	1 oz	80	3	4
Laughing Cow Babybel	1 oz	90	5	7
Marin French Cheese Camembert	1 oz	86	4	7
New Holland Havarti Lower Fat Garden Vegetable	1 oz	80	4	6
Polly-O Mozzarella Free	1 oz	35	0	0
Polly-O Mozzarella Lite	1 oz	60	2	3
Polly-O Mozzarella Part Skim	1 oz	70	3	5
Polly-O Mozzarella Whole Milk	1 oz	80	4	6
Polly-O Ricotta Free	¼ cup	50	0	0
Polly-O String Lite	1 stick (1 oz)	60	2	3
Sargento Blue Crumbled	¼ cup (1 oz)	100	5	8
Sargento Cheese For Nachos & Tacos Shredded	¼ cup (1 oz)	110	5	9
Sargento Jarlsberg	1 slice (1.2 oz)	120	5	9
Sargento Ricotta Light	¼ cup (2.2 oz)	60	2	3
Sargento Ricotta Part Skim	¼ cup (2.2 oz)	80	3	5
Treasure Cave Feta Crumbled	1 oz	80	4	6
Tree Of Life Cheddar 33% Reduced Fat Organic Milk	1 oz	90	4	6
Weight Watchers Fat Free Grated Parmesan	1 tbsp	15	0	0

CHEESE PROCESSED

FOOD	PORTION	CALS.	SAT. FAT	TOTAL FAT
Alouette Garlic	2 tbsp (0.8 oz)	70	5	7
Alouette Light Garlic	2 tbsp (0.8 oz)	50	3	4
Alpine Lace American	1 slice (0.66 oz)	50	2	3
Alpine Lace American Fat Free	1 piece (1 oz)	45	tr	tr
Borden Swiss Slices	1 oz	100	4	8
Cheez Whiz Light	2 tbsp (1.2 oz)	80	2	3
Cheez Whiz Spread	2 tbsp (1.2 oz)	90	5	7
Handi-Snacks Cheez'n Breadsticks	1 pkg (1.1 oz)	130	4	7
Harvest Moon American	1 slice (0.7 oz)	70	4	6

FOOD	PORTION	CALS.	SAT. FAT	TOTAL FAT
Healthy Choice American Singles White	1 slice (0.7 oz)	30	0	0
Heluva Good Cheese Cold Pack Cheddar Sharp With Jalapenos	2 tbsp (1 oz)	90	3	7
Kraft Deluxe Pimento	1 slice (1 oz)	100	6	8
Kraft Free Singles	1 slice (0.7 oz)	30	0	0
Kraft Free Singles Swiss	1 slice (0.7 oz)	30	0	0
Lactaid American	1 oz	94	4	7
Laughing Cow Assorted Wedge	1 (1 oz)	70	4	6
Laughing Cow Wedge Light	1 (1 oz)	50	2	3
Light N'Lively Singles 50% Less Fat American	0.7 oz	50	2	3
Old English American Sharp	1 oz	100	6	9
Price's Jalapeno Nacho Dip Mild	2 tbsp (1.1 oz)	80	3	7
Roka Spread Blue	2 tbsp (1.1 oz)	80	5	7
Rondele Light Soft Spreadable Garlic & Herb	2 tbsp (0.9 oz)	60	3	4
Rondele Soft Spreadable Garlic & Herbs	2 tbsp (1 oz)	100	6	9
Sargento MooTown Snackers Cheddar	1 piece (0.8 oz)	100	5	8
Smart Beat American	1 slice (0.6 oz)	35	1	2
Velveeta Cheese	1 slice (0.7 oz)	60	3	5
Velveeta Light	1 oz	60	2	3
Weight Watchers Fat Free Swiss	2 slices (0.75 oz)	30	0	0
WisPride Port Wine Ball	2 tbsp (1.1 oz)	100	4	8
WisPride Port Wine Light Cup	2 tbsp (1.1 oz)	80	2	3
CHEESE SUBSTITUTES				
Golden Image American	0.7 oz	70	2	5
Harvest Moon Cheddar Shredded	¼ cup (1.3 oz)	120	2	9
White Wave Soy A Melt Cheddar	1 oz	80	1	5
White Wave Soy A Melt Fat Free Cheddar	1 oz	40	0	tr
CHERRIES				
sweet fresh	10	49	tr	1
Sonoma Pitted Dried	¼ cup (1.4 oz)	140	0	0
CHESTNUTS				
roasted	2 to 3	70	tr	1

FOOD	PORTION	CALS.	SAT. FAT	TOTAL FAT
CHEWING GUM				
bubble gum	1 block (8 g)	27	0	0
stick	1 (3 g)	10	0	0
Chiclets Original	1 piece (1.59 g)	6	0	0
Trident Gum	1 piece (1.88 g)	5	0	0
CHICKEN				
breast & wing breaded & fried	2 pieces (5.7 oz)	494	8	30
broiler/fryer breast w/ skin batter dipped & fried	2.9 oz	218	3	11
broiler/fryer breast w/ skin roasted	½ breast (3.4 oz)	193	2	8
broiler/fryer breast w/o skin roasted	½ breast (3 oz)	142	1	3
broiler/fryer drumstick w/ skin batter dipped & fried	1 (2.6 oz)	193	3	11
broiler/fryer drumstick w/ skin roasted	1 (1.8 oz)	112	2	6
broiler/fryer drumstick w/o skin roasted	1 (1.5 oz)	76	1	2
cornish hen w/ skin roasted	1 hen (8 oz)	595	12	42
drumstick breaded & fried	2 pieces (5.2 oz)	430	7	27
nuggets breaded & fried w/ barbecue sauce	6 pieces (4.6 oz)	330	6	18
nuggets breaded & fried w/ sweet & sour sauce	6 pieces (4.6 oz)	346	6	18
oven roasted breast of chicken	½ breast	60	0	1
roaster light meat w/o skin roasted	1 cup (5 oz)	214	2	6
roaster w/ skin roasted	½ chicken (1.1 lbs)	1071	18	64
thigh breaded & fried	2 pieces (5.2 oz)	430	7	27
Banquet Breast Tenders Fat Free	3 (3.2 oz)	130	0	0
Banquet Country Fried frzn	1 serv (3 oz)	270	5	18
Banquet Nuggets frzn	3 oz	240	3	15
Banquet Wings Hot & Spicy frzn	4 pieces (5 oz)	230	5	16
Chicken By George Lemon Herb	1 breast (4 oz)	120	1	3
Country Skillet Chicken Patties frzn	2.5 oz	190	3	12
Empire Bologna	3 slices (1.8 oz)	200	2	7
Empire Stix frzn	4 (3.1 oz)	180	2	9
Healthy Choice Deli-Thin Oven Roasted Breast	6 slices (2 oz)	45	0	0

FOOD	PORTION	CALS.	SAT. FAT	TOTAL FAT
Hormel Chunk	2 oz	70	1	3
Oscar Mayer Lunchables Chicken/ Monterey Jack	1 pkg (4.5 oz)	350	10	21
Perdue Boneless Breasts Cooked	3 oz	120	1	2
Perdue Boneless Thighs Roasted	2 (3.5 oz)	200	3	11
Perdue Burger Cooked	1 (3 oz)	170	3	11
Perdue Chicken Breast Seasoned Barbecue Cooked	3 oz	110	1	1
Perdue Cornish Hen Split Dark Meat Roasted	½ hen (6.5 oz)	210	5	15
Perdue Drumsticks Roasted	1 (2 oz)	110	2	6
Perdue Oven Stuffer Dark Meat Roasted	3 oz	200	4	14
Perdue Oven Stuffer White Meat Roasted	3 oz	160	3	8
Perdue Short Cuts Mesquite	3 oz	110	1	2
Perdue Wingettes Roasted	3 (3 oz)	200	4	14
Perdue Wings Barbecued	3 oz	200	4	13
Tyson Roasted Drumsticks	2 (3.8 oz)	220	4	12

CHICKEN DISHES

FOOD	PORTION	CALS.	SAT. FAT	TOTAL FAT
chicken & noodles	1 cup	365	5	18
chicken cacciatore	¾ cup	394	6	24
chicken pie w/ top crust	1 slice (5.6 oz)	472	—	31
fillet sandwich plain	1	515	9	29
fillet sandwich w/ cheese lettuce mayonnaise & tomato	1	632	12	39
Croissant Pocket Stuffed Sandwich Chicken Broccoli & Cheddar	1 piece (4.5 oz)	300	4	11
Dinty Moore Chicken Stew	1 cup (7.5 oz)	180	2	8
Jimmy Dean Grilled Breast Sandwich	1 (5.5 oz)	330	4	11
Lean Pockets Stuffed Sandwich Chicken Fajita	1 (4.5 oz)	260	3	8
Weight Watchers Chicken Broccoli & Cheese Pocket Sandwich	1 (5 oz)	250	3	6

FOOD	PORTION	CALS.	SAT. FAT	TOTAL FAT
White Castle Grilled Chicken Sandwich	2 (4 oz)	250	3	9
CHICKEN SUBSTITUTES				
Soy Is Us Chicken Not!	½ cup (1.75 oz)	140	1	2
White Wave Meatless Sandwich Slices	2 slices (1.6 oz)	80	0	0
CHICKPEAS				
Old El Paso Garbanzo	½ cup (4.6 oz)	120	0	3
CHILI				
con carne w/ beans	1 cup	254	3	8
Gebhardt Plain	1 cup	530	16	43
Stouffer's With Beans	1 pkg (8.75 oz)	270	4	10
Tabatchnick Vegetarian	7.5 oz	210	1	6
CHIPS				
taro	10 (0.8 oz)	115	1	6
Barrel O' Fun Tortilla White	1 oz	140	—	6
Butterfield Potato Sticks	1 pkg (1.7 oz)	250	5	15
Eden Vegetable Chips	50 (1 oz)	130	2	4
Energy Food Factory Corn Pops Fat Free	½ oz	50	0	0
Energy Food Factory Potato Pops Fat Free	½ oz	50	0	0
Fritos Corn Chips	34 pieces (1 oz)	150	—	10
Kelly's Potato Rippled	1 oz	150	1	9
Louise's Potato Fat-Free Mesquite BBQ	1 oz	110	0	0
Louise's Potato Fat-Free No Salt	1 oz	110	0	0
Mr. Phipps Tater Crisps Original	23 (1 oz)	120	1	7
Mr. Phipps Tortilla Nacho	28 (1 oz)	130	1	4
Old El Paso Tortilla NACHIPS	9 chips (1 oz)	150	2	8
Pringles Potato Original	14 chips (1 oz)	160	3	11
State Line Potato	1 pkg (0.5 oz)	80	1	5
Terra Chips Sweet Potato	1 oz	140	1	7
Weight Watchers Potato Barbecue Curls	1 pkg (0.5 oz)	60	0	3
CHITTERLINGS				
pork simmered	3 oz	258	9	24

FOOD	PORTION	CALS.	SAT. FAT	TOTAL FAT
CHIVES				
fresh chopped	1 tbsp	1	tr	tr
CHOCOLATE				
chips milk chocolate	1 cup (3 oz)	431	15	26
chips semisweet	60 pieces (1 oz)	136	5	9
syrup	2 tbsp	82	tr	tr
syrup as prep w/ whole milk	9 oz	232	5	9
CHUTNEY				
tomato	1.2 oz	54	0	0
CILANTRO				
fresh	¼ cup	1	0	tr
CLAM JUICE				
Doxsee Canned	3 fl oz	4	0	0
CLAMS				
breaded & fried	20 sm	379	5	21
fresh cooked	20 sm	133	tr	2
fresh raw	9 lg (180 g)	133	tr	2
Gorton's Microwave Crunchy Clam Strips	3.5 oz	330	6	22
Progresso Minced	¼ cup (2 oz)	25	0	0
Progresso Red Clam Sauce	½ cup (4.4 oz)	80	1	3
Progresso White Clam Sauce	½ cup (4.4 oz)	120	2	9
COCOA				
Swiss Miss Hot Cocoa Milk Chocolate	1 serv	110	tr	1
Swiss Miss Hot Cocoa Sugar Free Milk Chocolate	1 serv	49	tr	tr
Swiss Miss Hot Cocoa Lite	1 serv	74	tr	tr
COCONUT				
cream canned	1 tbsp	36	3	3
dried sweetened flaked	¼ cup	88	5	6
fresh	1 piece (1.5 oz)	159	13	15
milk canned	½ cup	223	22	24
COD				
dried	3 oz	246	tr	2
fresh cooked	3 oz	89	tr	1
COFFEE				
brewed	6 oz	4	0	0

FOOD	PORTION	CALS.	SAT. FAT	TOTAL FAT
cafe au lait	1 cup (8 fl oz)	77	3	4
cafe brulot	1 cup (4.8 fl oz)	48	0	0
cappuccino	1 cup (8 fl oz)	77	3	4
coffee con leche	1 cup (8 fl oz)	77	3	4
espresso	1 cup (3 fl oz)	2	0	0
instant decaffeinated as prep	6 oz	4	0	0
instant regular	1 rounded tsp	4	0	0
instant regular w/ chickory as prep	6 oz	6	0	0
mocha	1 mug (9.6 fl oz)	202	9	15
COFFEE SUBSTITUTES				
Natural Touch Kaffree Roma	1 tsp	6	0	0
Postum Instant	6 oz	11	0	0
COFFEE WHITENERS				
Coffee-Mate Liquid	1 tbsp (0.5 fl oz)	16	tr	1
Coffee-Mate Powder	1 tsp (2 g)	10	1	1
International Delight Amaretto	1 tbsp (0.6 fl oz)	45	0	2
International Delight No Fat Amaretto	1 tbsp (0.5 fl oz)	30	0	0
Mocha Mix Fat-Free	1 tbsp (0.5 fl oz)	10	0	0
Mocha Mix Lite	1 tbsp (0.5 fl oz)	10	0	tr
Mocha Mix Original	1 tbsp (0.5 fl oz)	20	0	2
Mocha Mix Signature Flavors Irish Creme	1 tbsp (0.5 fl oz)	35	0	0
COLLARDS				
fresh cooked	½ cup	17	0	tr
COOKIES				
biscotti with nuts chocolate dipped	1 (1.3 oz)	117	3	6
Archway Almond Crescents	2 (0.8 oz)	100	1	4
Archway Chocolate Chip	1 (1 oz)	130	2	6
Archway Frosty Lemon	1 (1 oz)	120	1	5
Archway Pfeffernusse	2 (1.3 oz)	140	0	1
Bakery Wagon Cobbler Apple Fat Free	1	70	0	0
Baking On The Lite Side Oatmeal Crunchy	2 (0.6 oz)	60	0	0
Baking On The Lite Side Raspberry Linzer	1 (0.6 oz)	55	0	0
Barnum's Animal Crackers	12 (1.1 oz)	140	1	4

FOOD	PORTION	CALS.	SAT. FAT	TOTAL FAT
Biscos Sugar Wafers	8 (1 oz)	140	2	6
Chip-A-Roos Cookies	3 (1.3 oz)	190	4	10
Chips Ahoy! Reduced Fat	3 (1.1 oz)	150	2	6
Cookie Lover's Classic Shortbread	1 (0.8 oz)	110	2	7
Dutch Mill Coconut Macaroons	3 (1 oz)	120	6	7
Dutch Mill Oatmeal Raisin	3 (1 oz)	130	2	6
Estee Creme Wafers Lemon	5 (1.2 oz)	170	2	8
Frookie Animal Frackers	6	60	1	2
Golden Fruit Raisin	1 (0.7 oz)	80	0	2
Honey Maid Cinnamon Grahams	10 (1.1 oz)	140	1	3
Hydrox Original	3	150	2	7
Hydrox Reduced Fat	3 (1.1 oz)	130	1	4
Keebler Old Fashion Peanut Butter	1	80	1	4
Keebler Old Fashion Sugar	1	80	1	3
LU Le Petit Ecolier Dark Chocolate	2 (0.9 oz)	130	4	6
La Choy Fortune	1	15	—	tr
Little Debbie Oatmeal Lights	1 pkg (1.3 oz)	140	1	4
Little Debbie Peanut Butter	1 pkg (1.5 oz)	210	3	10
Lorna Doone Cookies	4 (1 oz)	140	1	7
Mallomars Cookies	2 (0.9 oz)	120	3	5
Manischewitz Macaroons Chocolate	2 (0.9 oz)	90	4	4
Mother's Macaroon	2	150	4	8
Mystic Mint Cookies	1 (0.5 oz)	90	1	4
Nabisco Brown Edge Wafers	5 (1 oz)	140	2	6
Nabisco Bugs Bunny Graham	13 (1.1 oz)	140	1	7
Nabisco Nilla Wafers	8 (1.1 oz)	140	1	5
National Arrowroot	1 (5 g)	20	0	1
Newtons Apple Fat Free	2 (1 oz)	100	0	0
Newtons Fig	2 (1.1 oz)	110	1	3
Newtons Fig Fat Free	1 (1 oz)	100	0	0
Nutter Butter Peanut Butter Sandwich	2 (1 oz)	130	1	6
Oreo Cookies	3 (1.2 oz)	160	2	7
Oreo Reduced Fat	3 (1.2 oz)	140	1	5
Pepperidge Farm Brussels	2	110	2	5
Pepperidge Farm Butter Chessman	2	90	2	4

FOOD	PORTION	CALS.	SAT. FAT	TOTAL FAT
Pepperidge Farm Fruit Filled Apricot-Raspberry	2	100	2	4
Pepperidge Farm Lemon Nut Crunch	2	110	2	7
Pepperidge Farm Pirouettes Chocolate Laced	2	70	1	4
Pepperidge Farm Ripple Milk Chocolate Fat Free	1 (0.6 oz)	60	0	0
SnackWell's Fat Free Cinnamon Grahams	20 (1 oz)	110	0	0
SnackWell's Fat Free Devil's Food	1 (0.5 oz)	50	0	0
SnackWell's Golden Devil's Food	1 (0.5 oz)	50	0	1
SnackWell's Reduced Fat Chocolate Chip	13 (1 oz)	130	2	4
SnackWell's Reduced Fat Chocolate Sandwich With Chocolate Creme	2 (0.9 oz)	100	1	3
SnackWell's Reduced Fat Vanilla Sandwich	2 (0.9 oz)	110	1	3
Social Tea Cookies	6 (1 oz)	120	1	4
Stella D'Oro Kichel Low Sodium	21	150	—	9
Sunshine Grahams Fudge Dipped	4 (1.2 oz)	170	6	9
Sunshine Vienna Fingers	2 (1 oz)	140	2	6
Tree Of Life Wheat-Free California Carob	1 (0.8 oz)	105	0	5
Vienna Fingers Low Fat	2 (1 oz)	130	1	4
Weight Watchers Apple Raisin Bar	1 (0.75 oz)	70	1	2
Weight Watchers Chocolate Chip	2 (1.06 oz)	140	2	5
Weight Watchers Fruit Filled Raspberry	1 (0.7 oz)	70	0	0

CORN

FOOD	PORTION	CALS.	SAT. FAT	TOTAL FAT
fritters	1 (1 oz)	62	tr	2
on-the-cob w/ butter cooked	1 ear	155	2	3
yellow cooked	1 ear (2.7 oz)	83	tr	1
Del Monte Cream Style Golden	½ cup (4.4 oz)	90	0	1
Green Giant In Butter Sauce frzn	½ cup	100	1	2
Green Giant Mexi Corn	½ cup	80	0	tr
Ka-Me Baby	½ cup (4.5 oz)	20	0	0

FOOD	PORTION	CALS.	SAT. FAT	TOTAL FAT
Stouffer's Souffle	½ cup (2.4 oz)	170	2	7
CORNMEAL				
hush puppies	1 (¾ oz)	74	tr	3
COTTAGE CHEESE				
Axelrod Nonfat	½ cup (4.4 oz)	90	0	0
Breakstone 2% Fat Large Curd	½ cup (4.2 oz)	90	2	3
Breakstone 4% Fat Large Curd	½ cup (4.2 oz)	120	4	5
Friendship Lowfat 1%	½ cup (4 oz)	90	1	1
Hood 1% Fat Chive & Onion	½ cup (4 oz)	90	1	2
Knudsen 1.5% Fat Pineapple	4 oz	110	1	2
Lactaid 1%	4 oz	72	1	1
Light N'Lively 1% Fat Garden Salad	½ cup (4.2 oz)	90	1	2
COUGH DROPS				
Halls Cough Drops	1 (3.8 g)	15	0	0
Lifesavers Menthol	2 (0.5 oz)	60	0	0
COUSCOUS				
cooked	½ cup	101	tr	tr
Casbah Pilaf as prep	1 cup	200	0	tr
CRAB				
alaska king cooked	1 leg (4.7 oz)	129	tr	2
baked	1 (3.8 oz)	160	tr	2
blue raw	1 crab (0.7 oz)	18	tr	tr
cake	1 (2 oz)	160	2	10
canned	½ cup	67	tr	1
soft-shell fried	1 (4.4 oz)	334	4	18
CRACKERS				
melba toast plain	1 (5 g)	19	tr	tr
saltines fat free low sodium	6 (1 oz)	118	tr	tr
Better Cheddars Crackers	22 (1 oz)	70	2	8
Better Cheddars Reduced Fat	24 (1 oz)	140	2	6
Burns & Ricker Bagel Crisps Garlic	5 (1 oz)	100	0	0
Cheez-It Crackers	27 (1 oz)	160	2	8
Cheez-It Reduced Fat	30 (1 oz)	130	1	5
Crown Pilot Crackers	1 (0.5 oz)	70	0	2
Eden Brown Rice	5 (1 oz)	120	0	2
Harvest Crisps 5 Grain	13 (1.1 oz)	130	1	4

FOOD	PORTION	CALS.	SAT. FAT	TOTAL FAT
Healthy Choice Bread Crisps Garlic Herb	11 (1 oz)	110	0	2
Hi Ho Crackers	9	160	2	9
Hi Ho Reduced Fat	10 (1.1 oz)	140	1	5
Ideal Crispbread Extra Thin	3	48	0	0
Keebler Club	2	30	tr	2
Lavash Bread Crisp Original	2 (0.5 oz)	60	tr	1
Little Debbie Cheese Crackers With Peanut Butter	1 pkg (1.4 oz)	210	3	10
Nabisco Swiss	15 (1 oz)	140	2	7
Nabisco Tid-Bit Cheese	32 (1 oz)	150	2	8
Nabisco Vegetable Thins	14 (1.1 oz)	160	2	9
Nabisco Wheat Thins Original	16 (1 oz)	140	1	6
Nabisco Wheat Thins Reduced Fat	18 (1 oz)	120	1	4
Oysterettes Crackers	19 (0.5 oz)	60	1	3
Partners Walla Walla Sweet Onion Preservative Free	0.5 oz	65	2	3
Pepperidge Farm Goldfish Cheddar Cheese	1 pkg (1.5 oz)	190	2	6
Planters Cheese Peanut Butter Sandwiches	1 pkg (1.4 oz)	190	2	10
Ritz Crackers	5 (0.5 oz)	80	1	4
Rykrisp Natural	2	40	0	0
Sesmark Brown Rice	15 (1 oz)	120	0	2
SnackWell's Cracked Pepper	7 (0.5 oz)	60	0	0
SnackWell's Fat Free Wheat	5 (0.5 oz)	60	0	0
SnackWell's Reduced Fat Cheese	38 (1 oz)	130	1	2
SnackWell's Reduced Fat Classic Golden	6 (0.5 oz)	60	0	1
SnackWell's Salsa Cheddar	32 (1 oz)	120	0	2
Tree Of Life Bite Size Fat Free Soya Nut	12	60	0	0
Triscuit Crackers	7 (1.1 oz)	140	1	5
Triscuit Reduced Fat	8 (1.1 oz)	130	1	3
Venus Armenian Thin Bread	2 (0.9 oz)	100	tr	1
Wasa Crispbread Extra Crisp	1	25	0	0
Wheatworth Stone Ground	5 (0.5 oz)	80	1	4
Zwieback Crackers	1 (8 g)	35	1	1

FOOD	PORTION	CALS.	SAT. FAT	TOTAL FAT
CRANBERRIES				
Ocean Spray Craisins	1/3 cup (1.4 oz)	130	0	0
Ocean Spray Cranberry Sauce Jellied	2 oz	90	0	0
Ocean Spray Whole Berry Sauce	2 oz	90	0	0
CRANBERRY JUICE				
After The Fall Cape Cod Cranberry	1 bottle (10 oz)	130	0	0
Ocean Spray Cocktail	8 fl oz	140	0	0
Ocean Spray Cocktail Reduced Calorie	8 fl oz	50	0	0
Snapple Cranberry Royal	10 fl oz	150	0	0
Tropicana Twister Ruby Red	1 bottle (10 fl oz)	150	0	0
CRAYFISH				
cooked	3 oz	97	tr	1
CREAM				
half & half	1 tbsp	20	1	2
whipped	1/4 cup	104	7	11
Farmland Light Cream	2 tbsp	30	2	3
CREAM CHEESE				
Alpine Lace Fat Free Garlic & Herbs	2 tbsp (1 oz)	30	tr	tr
Breakstone Temp-Tee Whipped	3 tbsp (1.2 oz)	110	7	10
Fleur De Lait Fresh Cut Garden Vegetable	2 tbsp (0.9 oz)	80	5	8
Healthy Choice Herbs & Garlic	2 tbsp (1 oz)	25	0	0
Philadelphia Free	1 oz	25	0	0
Philadelphia Light Soft	2 tbsp (1.1 oz)	70	4	5
Philadelphia Regular	1 oz	100	6	10
Philadelphia Whipped Smoked Salmon	3 tbsp (1.1 oz)	100	6	9
Weight Watchers Light	2 tbsp	40	2	3
CREAM CHEESE SUBSTITUTES				
Tofutti Better Than Cream Cheese Plain	1 oz	80	2	8
CROISSANT				
cheese	1 (2 oz)	236	5	12
plain	1 (2 oz)	232	7	12
w/ egg & cheese	1	369	14	25

FOOD	PORTION	CALS.	SAT. FAT	TOTAL FAT
w/ egg cheese & bacon	1	413	15	28
w/ egg cheese & ham	1	475	17	34
CROUTONS				
Arnold Crispy Cheese Garlic	½ oz	60	tr	2
CUCUMBER				
cucumber salad	½ cup	50	tr	tr
raw	1 (11 oz)	38	tr	tr
CUSTARD				
baked	½ cup (5 oz)	148	3	7
DANDELION GREENS				
fresh cooked	½ cup	17	0	tr
DANISH PASTRY				
cheese	1 (4¼ in) (2.5 oz)	266	5	16
cinnamon	1 (4¼ in) (2.3 oz)	262	4	15
cinnamon nut	1 (4¼ in) (2.3 oz)	280	4	16
fruit	1 (3.3 oz)	335	3	16
raisin	1 (4¼ in) (2.5 oz)	264	3	13
Morton Honey Buns	1 (2.28 oz)	250	3	10
DATES				
whole	5	114	0	tr
DELI MEATS/COLD CUTS				
blood sausage	1 oz	95	3	9
braunschweiger pork	1 oz	102	3	9
corned beef	2 oz	70	1	2
dried beef	1 oz	47	tr	1
mortadella beef & pork	1 oz	88	3	7
pepperoni pork & beef	1 slice (0.2 oz)	27	1	2
salami cooked beef & pork	1 oz	71	2	6
submarine w/ salami ham cheese lettuce tomato onion & oil	1	456	7	19
Healthy Choice Bologna	1 slice (1 oz)	30	0	1
Oscar Mayer Free Bologna	2 slices (1.6 oz)	35	0	0
Oscar Mayer Genoa Salami	3 slices (1 oz)	100	3	9
Russer Light Bologna	2 oz	120	4	8
Russer Light Braunschweiger	2 oz	120	3	8
Russer Olive Loaf	2 oz	160	5	13
Sara Lee Pastrami Beef	2 oz	100	3	6
Sara Lee Peppered Beef	2 oz	70	1	2

FOOD	PORTION	CALS.	SAT. FAT	TOTAL FAT
Spam Lite	2 oz	110	3	8
Spam Original	2 oz	170	6	16
DINNER				
Armour Classics Veal Parmigiana	1 meal (11.25 oz)	400	11	22
Armour Classics Lite Salisbury Steak	1 meal (11.5 oz)	260	4	7
Armour Classics Lite Shrimp Creole	1 meal (10 oz)	220	0	1
Banquet BBQ Style Chicken	1 meal (9 oz)	320	2	12
Banquet Chicken Parmigiana	1 pkg (9.5 oz)	290	4	15
Banquet Chicken Fried Steak	1 pkg (10 oz)	400	6	20
Banquet Extra Helping Meatloaf	1 meal (19 oz)	650	16	38
Banquet Family Entree Gravy & Sliced Turkey	1 serv (4.8 oz)	100	2	5
Banquet Hot Sandwich Toppers Chicken Ala King	1 pkg (4.5 oz)	100	2	4
Banquet Hot Sandwich Toppers Sloppy Joe	1 meal (4 oz)	140	3	7
Healthy Choice Beef & Peppers Cantonese	1 meal (11.5 oz)	270	3	5
Healthy Choice Chicken & Vegetables Marsala	1 meal (11.5 oz)	220	0	1
Healthy Choice Chicken Dijon	1 meal (11 oz)	280	2	4
Healthy Choice Classics Mesquite Beef Barbecue	1 meal (11 oz)	310	2	4
Healthy Choice Classics Shrimp & Vegetables Maria	1 meal (12.5 oz)	260	1	2
Healthy Choice Honey Mustard Chicken	1 meal (9.5 oz)	260	0	2
Healthy Choice Lemon Pepper Fish	1 meal (10.7 oz)	290	1	5
Healthy Choice Sweet & Sour Chicken	1 meal (11.5 oz)	310	1	5
Healthy Choice Traditional Beef Tips	1 meal (11.25 oz)	260	2	5
Kid Cuisine Chicken Sandwich	1 pkg (9.43 oz)	480	4	15
Life Choice Garden Potato Casserole	1 meal (13.4 oz)	160	0	1
Morton Breaded Chicken Pattie	1 meal (6.75 oz)	280	3	15

FOOD	PORTION	CALS.	SAT. FAT	TOTAL FAT
My Own Meal Beef Stew	1 pkg (10 oz)	260	3	11
My Own Meal Chicken Noodles	1 pkg (10 oz)	270	2	8
Stouffer's Stuffed Pepper	1 pkg (10 oz)	200	2	8
Weight Watchers Chicken Cordon Bleu	1 pkg (9 oz)	220	2	6
Weight Watchers Fried Filet Of Fish	1 pkg (7.7 oz)	230	3	8
Weight Watchers Roast Turkey Madallions	1 pkg (8.5 oz)	190	1	2
Weight Watchers Shrimp Marinara	1 pkg (9 oz)	190	1	2

DIP

FOOD	PORTION	CALS.	SAT. FAT	TOTAL FAT
Breakstone Sour Cream French Onion	2 tbsp (1.1 oz)	50	3	4
Chi-Chi's Fiesta Cheese	2 tbsp (0.9 oz)	40	1	3
Guiltless Gourmet Black Bean Mild	1 oz	25	0	0
Heluva Good Cheese Bacon Horseradish	2 tbsp (1.1 oz)	60	3	5
Knudsen Nacho Cheese	2 tbsp (1.1 oz)	60	3	4
Kraft Clam	2 tbsp (1.1 oz)	60	3	4
Kraft Ranch	2 tbsp (1.1 oz)	60	3	4
Louise's Fat Free Sour Cream & Onion	1 oz	25	0	0
Marzetti Blue Cheese Veggie	2 tbsp	200	4	21
Old El Paso Chunky Salsa Medium	2 tbsp (1 oz)	15	0	0
Snyder's Mustard Pretzel	2 tbsp (1.2 oz)	90	2	4

DOUGHNUTS

FOOD	PORTION	CALS.	SAT. FAT	TOTAL FAT
chocolate glazed	1 (1.5 oz)	175	3	8
creme filled	1 (3 oz)	307	6	21
french cruller glazed	1 (1.4 oz)	169	2	8
jelly	1 (3 oz)	289	4	16
Dutch Mill Donut Holes Double-Dipped Chocolate	3 (1.4 oz)	220	6	16
Freihofer's Assorted	1 (2 oz)	270	4	17
Hostess Crumb Regular	1 (1 oz)	130	4	8
Little Debbie Donut Sticks	1 pkg (1.6 oz)	210	3	13
Tastykake Plain	1 (47 g)	190	3	10

DRINK MIXERS

FOOD	PORTION	CALS.	SAT. FAT	TOTAL FAT
Bacardi Margarita Mix w/ rum	8 fl oz	160	0	0
Bacardi Pina Colada	8 fl oz	140	0	0

FOOD	PORTION	CALS.	SAT. FAT	TOTAL FAT
Libby Bloody Mary Mix	6 oz	40	0	0
DUCK				
w/ skin roasted	½ duck (13.4 oz)	1287	37	108
w/o skin roasted	½ duck (7.8 oz)	445	9	25
EEL				
fresh cooked	3 oz	200	3	13
smoked	3.5 oz	330	7	28
EGG				
fried w/ margarine	1	91	2	7
hard cooked	1	77	2	5
poached	1	74	2	5
scrambled plain	2	200	6	15
scrambled w/ whole milk & margarine	1	101	2	7
EGG DISHES				
deviled	2 halves	145	3	13
salad	½ cup	307	6	28
sandwich fried w/ cheese	1	340	7	19
sandwich fried w/ cheese & ham	1	348	7	16
EGG SUBSTITUTES				
Egg Beaters Eggs Substitute	¼ cup	25	0	0
Healthy Choice Cholesterol Free	¼ cup (2 oz)	25	0	0
Simply Eggs Egg Substitute	1.75 fl oz	35	tr	1
EGGNOG				
eggnog	1 cup	342	11	19
Hood Fat Free	4 fl oz	100	0	0
EGGPLANT				
baba ghannouj	¼ cup	55	—	4
caponata	2 tbsp (1 oz)	30	—	2
slices cooked	4 (7 oz)	38	0	0
ENDIVE				
raw chopped	½ cup	4	tr	tr
ENGLISH MUFFIN				
plain	1	134	tr	1
toasted w/ butter	1	189	2	6
toasted w/ egg cheese & canadian bacon	1	383	9	20
toasted w/ egg cheese & sausage	1	394	10	24

FOOD	PORTION	CALS.	SAT. FAT	TOTAL FAT
Thomas' Sandwich Size	1 (92 g)	210	1	2
FALAFEL				
falafel	1 (1.2 oz)	57	tr	3
FAVA BEANS				
Progresso Fava Beans	½ cup (4.6 oz)	110	0	1
FEIJOA				
fresh	1 (1.75 oz)	25	0	tr
FENNEL				
fresh sliced	1 cup	27	0	tr
FIGS				
fresh	1 med	50	tr	tr
Sonoma White Misson dried	3–4 (1.4 oz)	110	0	0
FISH				
breaded fillet frzn	1 (2 oz)	155	2	7
fish cake	1 (4.7 oz)	166	2	7
sandwich fried w/ tartar sauce	1	431	5	55
sandwich fried w/ tartar sauce & cheese	1	524	8	29
sticks frzn	1 stick (1 oz)	76	1	3
taramasalata	¼ cup	223	—	23
Port Clyde Fish Steaks In Mustard Sauce	1 can (3.75 oz)	140	1	7
Van De Kamp's Battered Fish Fillets	1 (2.6 oz)	180	2	11
Van De Kamp's Crisp & Healthy Breaded Fillets	2 (3.5 oz)	150	1	3
FLAN				
flan	½ cup (5.4 oz)	220	3	6
FLAXSEED				
Arrowhead Flaxseed	3 tbsp (1 oz)	140	1	10
FLOUNDER				
cooked	3 oz	99	tr	1
Van De Kamp's Lightly Breaded Fillets	1 (4 oz)	230	2	11
Van De Kamp's Natural Fillets	1 (4 oz)	110	0	2
FRENCH TOAST				
w/ butter	2 slices	356	8	19

FOOD	PORTION	CALS.	SAT. FAT	TOTAL FAT
FROG'S LEGS				
frog leg as prep w/ seasoned flour & fried	1 (0.8)	70	—	5
FRUIT DRINKS				
After The Fall Twist O' Strawberry	1 can (12 oz)	190	0	0
Hood Natural Blenders Apple Cranberry Raspberry	1 cup (8 oz)	130	0	0
Minute Maid Citrus Punch Chilled	8 fl oz	130	0	0
Ocean Spray Cranapple	8 fl oz	160	0	0
Ocean Spray Cranapple Reduced Calorie	8 fl oz	50	0	0
Odwalla Guanaba Dabba Doo!	8 fl oz	130	0	0
Pek Mango Guava Ecstasy	1 bottle (20 fl oz)	110	0	0
Snapple Diet Kiwi Strawberry	8 fl oz	13	0	0
FRUIT MIXED				
fruit cocktail juice pack	½ cup	56	tr	tr
fruit salad juice pack	½ cup	62	tr	tr
Del Monte Snack Cups Mixed Fruit Fruit Naturals EZ-Open Lid	1 serv (4.5 oz)	60	0	0
FRUIT SNACKS				
fruit leather rolls	1 lg (0.7 oz)	73	tr	1
Del Monte Sierra Trail Mix	¼ cup (1.2 oz)	150	3	8
Weight Watchers Apple Chips	1 pkg (0.75 oz)	70	0	0
GARLIC				
clove	1	4	tr	tr
GEFILTE FISH				
sweet	1 piece (1.5 oz)	35	tr	1
GELATIN				
Hunt's Snack Pack Juicy Gels Cherry	1 (4 oz)	100	0	0
GINGER				
Ka-Me Crystalized Slices	5 pieces (1 oz)	100	0	0
GOAT				
roasted	3 oz	122	1	3
GOOSE				
w/ skin roasted	6.6 oz	574	13	41
w/o skin roasted	5 oz	340	7	18

FOOD	PORTION	CALS.	SAT. FAT	TOTAL FAT
GRANOLA BARS				
chewy chocolate coated chocolate chip	1 (1 oz)	132	4	7
chewy chocolate coated peanut butter	1 (1 oz)	144	5	9
chewy raisin	1 (1 oz)	127	3	5
plain	1 (1 oz)	134	1	7
Kellogg's Low Fat Crunchy Cinnamon Raisin	1 (0.7 oz)	80	0	2
GRANOLA CEREAL				
granola	¼ cup	138	1	8
Grist Mill Low-Fat With Raisins	⅔ cup (1.9 oz)	220	1	3
Uncle Roy's Organic Golden Honey	½ cup (1.6 oz)	190	1	6
GRAPE JUICE				
Minute Maid Chilled	8 fl oz	130	0	0
Seneca White Grape Juice frzn as prep	8 fl oz	140	0	0
GRAPE LEAVES				
Cedar's Grape Leaves Stuffed With Rice	6 pieces (4.9 oz)	180	1	8
GRAPEFRUIT				
pink	½	37	tr	tr
red	½	37	tr	tr
white	½	39	tr	tr
S&W Sections In Light Syrup	½ cup	80	0	0
GRAPEFRUIT JUICE				
fresh	1 cup	96	tr	tr
frzn as prep	1 cup	102	tr	tr
GRAPES				
grapes	10	36	tr	tr
GRAVY				
beef	¼ cup	31	tr	1
GREAT NORTHERN BEANS				
canned	1 cup	150	0	tr
GREEN BEANS				
canned	½ cup	13	tr	tr
cooked	½ cup	22	tr	tr
Green Giant Almondine	½ cup	45	0	3

FOOD	PORTION	CALS.	SAT. FAT	TOTAL FAT
Stouffer's Green Bean Mushroom Casserole	½ cup (1.9 oz)	130	2	8
GUAVA				
fresh	1	45	tr	1
Kern's Nectar	6 fl oz	110	0	0
HADDOCK				
cooked	3 oz	95	tr	1
smoked	1 oz	33	tr	tr
Van De Kamp's Battered Fillets	2 (4 oz)	260	3	16
Van De Kamp's Lightly Breaded Fillets	1 (4 oz)	220	2	10
HALIBUT				
cooked	3 oz	119	tr	2
HAM				
Alpine Lace Boneless Cooked	2 oz	60	1	2
Healthy Choice Deli-Thin Honey With Natural Juices	6 slices (2 oz)	60	1	2
Hormel Deviled Ham	4 tbsp (2 oz)	150	4	12
Oscar Mayer Dinner Slice	3 oz	90	1	3
Oscar Mayer Dinner Steaks	1 (2 oz)	60	1	2
Russer Chopped	2 oz	130	3	9
Sara Lee Honey Roasted	2 oz	90	2	5
Underwood Deviled Light	2.08 oz	120	1	8
HAM DISHES				
croquettes	1 (3.1 oz)	217	5	14
salad	½ cup	287	5	23
sandwich w/ cheese	1	353	6	15
Weight Watchers Ham & Cheese Pocket Sandwich	1 (5 oz)	240	3	7
HAMBURGER				
double patty w/ bun	1 reg	544	10	28
double patty w/ ketchup cheese mayonnaise mustard pickle tomato & bun	1 lg	706	18	44
single patty w/ bacon ketchup cheese mustard onion pickle & bun	1 lg	609	16	37
single patty w/ bun	1 reg	275	4	12

FOOD	PORTION	CALS.	SAT. FAT	TOTAL FAT
single patty w/ bun	1 lg	400	8	23
single patty w/ cheese & bun	1 lg	608	15	33
Kid Cuisine Beef Patty Sandwich w/ Cheese	1 (8.5 oz)	410	5	15
White Castle Cheeseburger	2 (3.6 oz)	310	9	17
HEARTS OF PALM				
canned	1 (1.2 oz)	9	tr	tr
HERRING				
fresh cooked	3 oz	172	2	10
kippered	1 fillet (1.4 oz)	87	1	5
pickled	½ oz	39	tr	3
HOMINY				
Van Camp's White	½ cup (4.3 oz)	80	0	1
HONEY				
honey	1 tbsp (0.7 oz)	64	0	0
HONEYDEW				
wedge	1/10	46	0	tr
HORSERADISH				
Hebrew National White	1 tbsp	7	0	0
Kraft Horseradish Mustard	1 tsp (0.2 oz)	0	0	0
Rosoff's Red	1 tbsp (0.5 oz)	8	0	0
HOT DOG				
corn dog	1	460	5	19
w/ bun chili	1	297	5	13
w/ bun plain	1	242	5	15
Empire Chicken	1 (2 oz)	100	2	7
Healthy Choice Beef	1 (1.8 oz)	60	1	2
Louis Rich Bun Length Turkey	1 (2 oz)	110	3	8
Oscar Mayer Free	1 (1.8 oz)	40	0	0
Shofar Kosher Beef Reduced Fat Reduced Sodium	1 (1.8 oz)	120	4	10
HUMMUS				
hummus	1/3 cup	140	1	7
ICE CREAM AND FROZEN DESSERTS				
cone vanilla light soft serve	1 (4.6 oz)	164	4	6
dixie cup chocolate	1 (3.5 fl oz)	125	4	6
dixie cup vanilla	1 (3.5 fl oz)	116	4	6

FOOD	PORTION	CALS.	SAT. FAT	TOTAL FAT
freeze dried ice cream chocolate strawberry & vanilla	1 pkg (0.75 oz)	158	2	5
gelato chocolate hazelnut	½ cup (5.3 oz)	370	4	29
gelato vanilla	½ cup (3 oz)	211	8	15
Ben & Jerry's Cherry Garcia	½ cup (3.7 oz)	240	10	16
Ben & Jerry's Chunky Monkey	½ cup (3.7 oz)	280	10	19
Ben & Jerry's New York Super Fudge Chunk	½ cup (3.7 oz)	290	11	20
Ben & Jerry's No Fat Vanilla Fudge Swirl	½ cup (3.1 oz)	150	0	0
Ben & Jerry's Rain Forest Crunch	½ cup (3.7 oz)	300	11	23
DoveBar Vanilla Milk Chocolate	1 (3.8 fl oz)	340	13	21
Drumstick Cone Chocolate Dipped	1 (4.6 oz)	340	10	17
Friendly's Heath English Toffee	½ cup (2.7 oz)	190	6	10
Friendly's Purely Pistachio	½ cup	160	6	10
Haagen-Dazs Butter Pecan	½ cup (3.7 oz)	320	11	24
Haagen-Dazs Cappuccino Commotion	½ cup (3.6 oz)	310	12	21
Haagen-Dazs Cookies & Cream	½ cup (3.6 oz)	270	11	17
Haagen-Dazs Vanilla	½ cup (3.7 oz)	270	11	18
Healthy Choice Fudge Brownie	½ cup (2.5 oz)	120	1	2
Healthy Choice Mint Chocolate Chip	½ cup (2.5 oz)	120	1	2
Healthy Choice Rocky Road	½ cup (2.5 oz)	140	1	2
Hood Chocolate	½ cup (2.3 oz)	140	5	7
Hood Coffee	½ cup (2.3 oz)	140	5	7
Hood Fat Free Heavenly Hash	½ cup (2.5 oz)	120	0	0
Hood Fat Free Very Vanilla	½ cup (2.5 oz)	100	0	0
Hood Light Heavenly Hash	½ cup (2.4 oz)	130	2	4
Hood Light Vanilla Chocolate Strawberry	½ cup (2.4 oz)	110	2	4
Hood Spumoni	½ cup (2.3 oz)	140	5	9
Hood Strawberry	½ cup (2.3 oz)	130	5	7
Starbucks Frappuccino	1 bar (2.8 oz)	110	1	2
Turkey Hill Black Cherry	½ cup (2.3 oz)	140	5	7
Turkey Hill Lite Butter Pecan	½ cup (2.3 oz)	130	3	6
Turkey Hill Lite Vanilla Bean	½ cup (2.3 oz)	110	2	3
Weight Watchers Caramel Nut Bars	1 bar	130	4	8

FOOD	PORTION	CALS.	SAT. FAT	TOTAL FAT
Weight Watchers Chocolate Dip	1 bar	100	3	6
Weight Watchers English Toffee Crunch Bars	1 bar	120	4	7
Weight Watchers Vanilla Sandwich	1 bar	160	2	4
ICE CREAM TOPPINGS				
butterscotch	2 tbsp (1.4 oz)	103	tr	tr
caramel	2 tbsp (1.4 oz)	103	tr	tr
marshmallow cream	2 tbsp	88	0	tr
strawberry	2 tbsp (1.5 oz)	107	0	tr
walnuts in syrup	2 tbsp (1.4 oz)	167	1	9
ICED TEA				
Arizona Raspberry	8 fl oz	95	0	0
Crystal Light Decaffeinated Sugar Free	8 oz	2	0	0
Lipton Chilled Diet Lemon	8 fl oz	0	0	0
Lipton Chilled Lemon	8 fl oz	80	0	0
Royal Mistic Lemon	12 fl oz	144	0	0
Snapple Lemon	8 fl oz	110	0	0
Turkey Hill Regular	1 cup (8 oz)	90	0	0
ICES AND ICE POPS				
ice pop	1 (2 fl oz)	42	0	0
Dole Fruit 'N Juice Lemonade	1 bar (4 oz)	120	0	0
Frozfruit Strawberry	1 (4 oz)	80	0	0
Good Humor Creamsicle Orange	1 (1.8 fl oz)	70	1	2
Good Humor Fudgsicle Pop	1 (1.8 fl oz)	60	1	1
Haagen-Dazs Sorbet Chocolate	½ cup (4 oz)	130	0	0
Haagen-Dazs Sorbet Zesty Lemon	½ cup (4 oz)	130	0	0
Tofutti Frutti Apricot Mango	4 fl oz	100	0	0
JAM/JELLY/PRESERVES				
all flavors jam	1 pkg (0.5 oz)	34	0	0
all flavors jelly	1 pkg (0.5 oz)	38	0	0
all flavors preserve	1 pkg (0.5 oz)	34	0	0
apple butter	1 tbsp (0.6 oz)	33	0	0
orange marmalade	1 pkg (0.5 oz)	34	0	0
Smucker's All Flavors Simply Fruit	1 tsp	16	0	0
KALE				
chopped cooked	½ cup	21	tr	tr

FOOD	PORTION	CALS.	SAT. FAT	TOTAL FAT
KETCHUP				
Heinz Lite	1 tbsp	8	0	0
Hunt's Regular	1 tbsp (0.6 oz)	16	0	tr
Tree Of Life Salsa Ketchup	1 tbsp (0.5 oz)	10	0	0
KIDNEY BEANS				
Green Giant Dark Red	½ cup	90	0	0
KIWIS				
fresh	1 med	46	0	tr
KNISH				
potato	1 lg (7 oz)	332	3	12
KOHLRABI				
raw sliced	½ cup	19	tr	tr
sliced cooked	½ cup	24	tr	tr
KUMQUATS				
fresh	1	12	0	tr
LAMB				
cubed lean only broiled	3 oz	158	2	6
ground broiled	3 oz	240	7	17
leg roast lean & fat Choice roasted	3 oz	219	6	14
loin chop w/ bone lean & fat Choice broiled	1 chop (2.3 oz)	201	6	15
rib chop lean & fat Choice broiled	3 oz	307	11	25
shank lean & fat Choice braised	3 oz	206	5	11
LAMB DISHES				
curry	¾ cup	345	3	17
moussaka	5.6 oz	312	—	21
LEEKS				
chopped cooked	¼ cup	8	tr	tr
LEMON				
wedge	1	5	tr	tr
LEMON JUICE				
Realemon Juice	1 fl oz	6	0	0
LEMONADE				
4C Instant as prep	8 fl oz	80	0	0
After The Fall Apple Raspberry	1 bottle (10 oz)	120	0	0
Country Time Mix	8 fl oz	82	0	0
Fruitopia Lemonade	8 fl oz	120	0	0

FOOD	PORTION	CALS.	SAT. FAT	TOTAL FAT
Minute Maid Pink frzn	8 fl oz	120	0	0
Newman's Own Roadside Virginia	8 fl oz	100	0	tr
Royal Mistic Lemonade Limeade	16 fl oz	230	0	0
Snapple Diet Pink	8 fl oz	13	0	0
Tropicana Lemonade	1 can (11.5 oz)	160	0	0
LENTILS				
cooked	1 cup	231	tr	1
Casbah Pilaf as prep	1 cup	200	0	tr
LETTUCE				
bibb	½ head (3 oz)	11	tr	tr
boston	2 leaves	2	tr	tr
iceberg	1 leaf	3	tr	tr
romaine shredded	½ cup	4	tr	tr
LIMA BEANS				
Birds Eye Baby	½ cup	130	0	0
Del Monte Green	½ cup (4.4 oz)	80	0	0
LIME				
wedge	1	3	0	tr
LIME JUICE				
Odwalla Summertime Lime	8 fl oz	90	0	0
Realime Juice	1 oz	6	0	0
LIQUOR/LIQUEUR				
anisette	⅔ oz	74	0	0
apricot brandy	⅔ oz	64	0	0
benedictine	⅔ oz	69	0	0
bloody mary	5 oz	116	0	tr
bourbon & soda	4 oz	105	0	0
coffee liqueur	1½ oz	174	tr	tr
coffee w/ cream liqueur	1½ oz	154	5	7
creme de menthe	1½ oz	186	tr	tr
curacao liqueur	⅔ oz	54	0	0
daiquiri frzn	1 serv	111	0	0
gin	1½ oz	110	0	0
manhattan	2 oz	128	0	0
martini	2½ oz	156	0	0
pina colada	4½ oz	262	1	3
rum	1½ oz	97	0	0
sloe gin fizz	2½ oz	132	0	0

FOOD	PORTION	CALS.	SAT. FAT	TOTAL FAT
tequila sunrise	5½ oz	189	tr	tr
vodka	1½ oz	97	0	0
whiskey sour	3 oz	123	tr	tr
LIVER				
beef pan-fried	3 oz	184	2	7
chicken stewed	1 cup (5 oz)	219	3	8
LOBSTER				
cooked	3 oz	83	tr	1
newburg	1 cup	485	—	27
LOTUS				
root sliced cooked	10 slices	59	tr	tr
LYCHEES				
fresh	1	6	0	tr
Ka-Me Whole Pitted In Syrup	15 pieces (5 oz)	130	0	0
MACADAMIA NUTS				
oil roasted	1 oz	204	3	22
Mauna Loa Chocolate Covered	1 oz	170	—	13
MACKEREL				
canned	1 can (12.7 oz)	563	7	23
cooked	3 oz	223	4	15
MALT				
nonalcoholic	12 fl oz	32	0	0
Bartles & Jaymes Malt Cooler Original	12 fl oz	180	0	0
Olde English Malt	12 oz	163	0	0
MALTED MILK				
chocolate as prep w/ milk	1 cup	229	6	9
Kraft Instant Natural as prep w/ 2% milk	1 serv (9.5 oz)	210	4	7
MANGO				
fresh	1	135	tr	1
Sonoma Dried Pieces	8 pieces (2 oz)	180	0	1
MANGO JUICE				
Libby Nectar	1 can (11.5 fl oz)	210	0	0
Snapple Diet Mango Madness	8 fl oz	13	0	0
Snapple Mango Madness Cocktail	8 fl oz	110	0	0

FOOD	PORTION	CALS.	SAT. FAT	TOTAL FAT
MARGARINE				
squeeze	1 tsp	34	1	4
stick	1 tsp	34	1	4
tub	1 tsp	34	1	4
tub diet	1 tsp	17	tr	2
MARSHMALLOW				
Campfire Large	2	40	0	0
Campfire Miniature	24	40	0	0
Joyva Twists Chocolate Covered	2 (1.5 oz)	190	2	4
Kraft Marshmallow Creme	2 tbsp (0.4 oz)	40	0	0
MATZO				
egg	1 (1 oz)	111	tr	1
Horowitz Margareten Egg Milk Chocolate Coated	1 oz	97	3	4
Manischewitz Matzo Cracker Miniatures	10	90	0	tr
Manischewitz Plain	1	110	0	tr
Streit's Whole Wheat	1 (1 oz)	110	0	1
MAYONNAISE				
Best Foods Light	1 tbsp (15 g)	50	1	5
Best Foods Real	1 tbsp	100	2	11
Hain Eggless No Salt Added	1 tbsp	110	2	12
Hellman's Light Reduced Calorie	1 tbsp (15 g)	50	1	5
Kraft Free	1 tbsp (0.6 oz)	10	0	0
Kraft Light	1 tbsp (0.5 oz)	50	1	5
Kraft Real	1 tbsp (0.5 oz)	100	2	11
Smart Beat Canola Oil	1 tbsp	40	tr	4
Weight Watchers Fat Free	1 tbsp	10	0	0
MAYONNAISE TYPE SALAD DRESSING				
Miracle Whip Free	1 tbsp (0.6 oz)	15	0	0
Miracle Whip Light	1 tbsp (0.5 oz)	40	0	3
Miracle Whip Regular	1 tbsp (0.5 oz)	70	1	7
Weight Watchers Fat Free Whipped Dressing	1 tbsp	15	0	0
MEAT STICKS				
Tombstone Beef Jerky	1 stick (0.5 oz)	35	0	0
Tombstone Beef Sticks	1 (0.8 oz)	110	5	10

FOOD	PORTION	CALS.	SAT. FAT	TOTAL FAT
MEAT SUBSTITUTES				
Boca Burgers Original	1 patty (2.5 oz)	110	1	2
Green Giant Harvest Burgers Original	1 (3 oz)	140	2	4
Ken & Robert's Veggie Burger	1 (62 g)	110	0	2
Lightlife Smart Deli Slices	2 slices (1.5 oz)	44	0	0
Lightlife Smart Dogs	1 (1.5 oz)	40	0	0
Morningstar Farms Garden Grain Patties	1 patty (2.5 oz)	120	1	3
Soy Is Us Beef Not!	½ cup (1.75 oz)	140	1	2
White Wave Meatless Healthy Franks	1 (1.5 oz)	90	0	2
White Wave Veggie Burger	1 patty (2.5 oz)	110	0	3
MILK				
1%	1 cup	102	2	3
2%	1 cup	121	3	5
buttermilk	1 cup	99	1	2
goat	1 cup	168	7	10
skim	1 cup	86	tr	tr
whole	1 cup	150	5	8
Calcimilk	8 fl oz	102	2	3
Carnation Evaporated	2 tbsp	40	2	3
Carnation Evaporated Lowfat	2 tbsp	25	tr	1
Carnation Sweetened Condensed	2 tbsp	130	2	3
Lactaid Nonfat	8 fl oz	86	tr	tr
Parmalat 2%	1 cup (8 oz)	130	3	5
MILK DRINKS				
Body Wise Chocolate Nonfat Milk	1 cup (8 fl oz)	180	0	0
Hood Chocolate Lowfat	1 cup (8 oz)	150	1	2
Parmalat Chocolate 2%	1 box (8 oz)	180	3	5
MILK SUBSTITUTES				
Eden Original	1 pkg (8.8 oz)	135	1	4
EdenRice Milk	8 fl oz	110	1	3
Edensoy Carob	8 fl oz	150	1	4
Edensoy Extra Vanilla	1 pkg (8.8 fl oz)	150	0	3
Vitasoy Original Light	8 fl oz	90	1	2
Westsoy Cocoa Lite	8 fl oz	140	tr	2

FOOD	PORTION	CALS.	SAT. FAT	TOTAL FAT
MILKSHAKE				
thick shake chocolate	10.6 oz	356	5	8
thick shake vanilla	11 oz	350	6	10
Hood Shake Up Strawberry	1 cup (8 oz)	220	3	5
Parmalat Shake A Shake Orange Vanilla	1 box (6 oz)	110	2	3
Weight Watchers Chocolate Fudge Shake Mix as prep	1 pkg	80	0	1
MINERAL/BOTTLED WATER				
Canada Dry Sparkling Water	8 fl oz	0	0	0
Crystal Geyser Sparkling Orange	1 bottle (12 fl oz)	0	0	0
Evian Water	1 liter	0	0	0
San Pellegrino Mineral Water	1 liter (33.8 oz)	0	0	0
Saratoga Sparkling	1 liter	0	0	0
MOLASSES				
Brer Rabbit Dark	2 tbsp	110	0	0
Tree Of Life Blackstrap	1 tbsp (0.5 oz)	45	0	0
MOUSSE				
chocolate	½ cup (7.1 oz)	447	19	33
Weight Watchers Triple Chocolate Caramel Mousse	1 (2.75 oz)	200	1	4
MUFFIN				
blueberry	1 (2 oz)	165	1	6
toaster type corn	1	114	1	4
Dutch Mill Carrot	1 (2 oz)	190	2	7
Hostess Mini Apple Cinnamon	5 (2 oz)	260	3	16
Pepperidge Farm Corn	1	180	1	7
Weight Watchers Banana Nut	1 (2.5 oz)	190	2	3
MUNG BEANS				
stir fried	½ cup	31	tr	tr
MUSHROOMS				
chanterelle	3½ oz	11	0	tr
enoki raw	1 (4 in)	2	tr	tr
morel	3½ oz	9	0	tr
oyster	3.5 oz	11	0	tr
raw sliced	½ cup	9	tr	tr
shiitake cooked	4 (2.5 oz)	40	tr	tr
sliced cooked	½ cup	21	tr	tr

FOOD	PORTION	CALS.	SAT. FAT	TOTAL FAT
Empire Breaded frzn	7 (2.8 oz)	90	0	1
Green Giant Oriental Straw	¼ cup	12	0	0
MUSSELS				
cooked	3 oz	147	1	4
MUSTARD				
Eden Hot Organic	1 tsp (5 g)	0	0	0
Grey Poupon Country Dijon	1 tsp	6	0	0
Gulden's Mild	1 tsp	6	0	0
Heinz Spicy Brown	1 tbsp	14	0	1
McIlhenny Coarse Ground	1 tsp (0.2 oz)	4	tr	tr
Plochman Squeeze Salad	1 tsp (5 g)	4	0	tr
Russer Deli	1 tsp (5 g)	4	0	0
Watkins Horseradish	1 tsp (7 oz)	10	0	0
MUSTARD GREENS				
chopped cooked	½ cup	11	tr	tr
NAVY BEANS				
Allen Navy Beans	½ cup (4.5 oz)	110	0	1
Trappey With Bacon & Jalapeno	½ cup (4.5 oz)	110	1	2
NECTARINE				
fresh	1	67	0	1
NEUFCHATEL				
Philadelphia Neufchatel	1 oz	70	4	6
Spreadery Garden Vegetable	2 tbsp (1 oz)	70	4	6
NOODLE DISHES				
noodle pudding	½ cup	132	4	7
Dinty Moore Noodles & Chicken	1 can (7.5 oz)	180	2	8
La Choy Ramen Noodles Chicken as prep	1 cup	200	1	7
Lipton Noodles & Sauce Cheese	⅔ cup (2.3 oz)	250	2	5
Minute Microwave Chicken Flavored	½ cup	157	2	5
NOODLES				
egg cooked	1 cup	212	tr	2
japanese soba cooked	½ cup	56	tr	tr
japanese somen cooked	½ cup	115	tr	tr
spinach/egg cooked	1 cup	211	tr	3
Golden Grain Egg	2 oz	210	1	2
Herb's Kluski	2 oz	220	0	2

FOOD	PORTION	CALS.	SAT. FAT	TOTAL FAT
Hodgson Mill Whole Wheat Egg	2 oz	190	1	2
Ka-Me Lo Mein Wide Chinese	½ cup (2 oz)	200	0	0
Ka-Me Py Mai Fun Rice Sticks	2 oz	193	0	0
Ka-Me Sai Fun Bean Thread	1 cup (2 oz)	190	0	0
Ka-Me Udon Japanese Thick	2 oz	190	0	1
La Choy Chow Mein Wide	½ cup	150	1	8
Shofar No Yolks	2 oz	210	0	0
NUTRITIONAL SUPPLEMENTS				
Boost Chocolate	1 can (8 oz)	240	1	4
Gatorade GatorBar	1 (1.17 oz)	110	0	1
Gatorade GatorLode	1 can (11.6 fl oz)	280	0	0
Gatorade GatorPro	1 can (11 fl oz)	360	1	6
Gatorade ReLode	1 pkt (0.75 oz)	80	0	0
Meal On The Go Original	1 bar (3 oz)	286	2	9
Sustacal Vanilla	8 oz	240	1	6
Vita-J Fruit Punch	11.5 fl oz	8	0	0
NUTS MIXED				
Fisher Mixed Deluxe Lightly Salted	1 oz	180	3	16
Fisher Nut & Fruit Tropical Fruit	1 oz	140	1	8
Planters Cashews & Peanuts Honey Roasted	1 oz	150	2	12
OCTOPUS				
fresh steamed	3 oz	140	tr	2
OIL				
cod liver	1 tbsp	123	3	14
wheat germ	1 tbsp	120	3	14
Eden Hot Pepper Sesame	1 tbsp (0.5 oz)	130	2	14
Hain Garlic & Oil	1 tbsp	120	3	14
Hain Walnut	1 tbsp	120	2	14
House Of Tsang Hot Chili Sesame	1 tsp (5 g)	45	1	5
Italica Olive Oil	1 tbsp	120	2	9
Mazola No Stick	2.5 second spray (0.2 g)	2	tr	tr
Pam Cooking Spray	1 second spray (0.266 g)	2	—	tr
Pam Olive Oil	1 second spray (0.266 g)	2	—	tr
Planters Popcorn	1 tbsp (0.5 oz)	120	3	14

FOOD	PORTION	CALS.	SAT. FAT	TOTAL FAT
Wesson Corn	1 tbsp	120	2	14
OKRA				
sliced cooked	½ cup	25	tr	tr
McIlhenny Pickled	2 pieces (1 oz)	7	tr	tr
Trappey Creole Gumbo	½ cup (4.2 oz)	35	0	0
OLIVES				
green	3 extra lg	15	tr	2
ripe	1 lg	5	tr	tr
Progresso Oil Cured	6 (0.5 oz)	80	1	6
Progresso Olive Salad (drained)	2 tbsp (0.8 oz)	25	0	3
ONION				
chopped cooked	½ cup	47	tr	tr
fried	¼ cup	88	3	6
raw chopped	1 tbsp	4	tr	tr
rings breaded & fried	8 to 9	275	7	16
scallions raw chopped	1 tbsp	2	tr	tr
Antioch Farms Vidalia	1 med	60	0	0
Birds Eye Small With Cream Sauce	½ cup	100	1	3
Vlasic Lightly Spiced Cocktail Onions	1 oz	4	0	0
ORANGE				
california navel	1	65	tr	tr
california valencia	1	59	tr	tr
florida	1	69	tr	tr
sections	1 cup	85	tr	tr
Empress Mandarin	5.5 oz	100	0	0
ORANGE JUICE				
chilled	1 cup	110	tr	1
fresh	1 cup	111	tr	tr
frzn as prep	1 cup	112	tr	tr
Hi-C Box	8.45 fl oz	130	0	0
Hood With Calcium	1 cup (8 oz)	120	0	0
Minute Maid Country Style Chilled	8 fl oz	110	0	0
Snapple Orangeade	8 fl oz	120	0	0
Tang Breakfast Crystals as prep	6 oz	86	0	0
Tropicana Juice	1 container (8 fl oz)	110	0	0
ORIENTAL FOOD				
chicken teriyaki w/ rice	1 serv (11 oz)	430	1	6

FOOD	PORTION	CALS.	SAT. FAT	TOTAL FAT
chop suey w/ pork	1 cup	375	8	29
chow mein chicken	1 cup	255	4	10
chow mein shrimp	1 cup	221	1	10
chow mein vegetable	1 serv (8 oz)	90	0	3
egg roll meat & shrimp	1 (4.8 oz)	320	3	12
egg roll shrimp	1 (3 oz)	170	1	5
egg roll vegetable	1 (3 oz)	170	1	4
fried rice	1 cup	249	—	6
oriental pepper & beef	1 serv (8 oz)	90	0	0
spring roll deep fried	1	202	—	9
sweet & sour pork	1 serv (8 oz)	250	3	8
wonton fried	½ cup (1 oz)	111	1	8
wonton soup	1 cup	205	1	3
Chun King Eggrolls Mini Chicken	8 (4.4 oz)	270	2	9
La Choy Dinner Classics Egg Foo Young	2 patties + 3 oz sauce	170	2	7
La Choy Dinner Classics Sweet & Sour	¾ cup	310	1	6
Luigino's Lo Mein Shrimp	1 pkg (8 oz)	190	1	3
Luigino's Szechwan Vegetable	1 pkg (6 oz)	350	4	12
OYSTERS				
battered & fried	6 (4.9 oz)	368	5	18
fresh cooked	6 med	58	1	2
fresh raw	6 med	58	1	2
stew	1 cup	278	10	18
Bumble Bee Whole Canned	½ cup (3.5 oz)	100	1	4
PANCAKE/WAFFLE SYRUP				
Aunt Jemima Lite	¼ cup (2.5 oz)	100	0	0
Aunt Jemima Regular	¼ cup (2.8 oz)	210	0	0
Tree Of Life Maple	¼ cup (2.1 oz)	200	0	0
PANCAKES				
buckwheat	1 (4 in diam)	55	1	2
potato	1 (4 in diam)	78	1	6
w/ butter & syrup	3	519	6	14
Aunt Jemima Lowfat	3 (3.4 oz)	130	0	2
Aunt Jemima Original	3 (3.4 oz)	200	1	3
PAPAYA				
cubed	1 cup	54	tr	tr

FOOD	PORTION	CALS.	SAT. FAT	TOTAL FAT
Goya Nectar	6 oz	110	0	0
Sonoma Pieces Dried	2 pieces (2 oz)	200	0	4
PARSLEY				
Dole Chopped	1 tbsp	10	0	tr
PARSNIPS				
fresh sliced cooked	½ cup	63	tr	tr
PASSION FRUIT JUICE				
purple	1 cup	126	0	tr
yellow	1 cup	149	0	tr
PASTA				
elbows cooked	1 cup	197	tr	tr
protein fortified cooked	1 cup	188	tr	tr
shells cooked	1 cup	197	tr	tr
spaghetti cooked	1 cup	197	tr	tr
spinach spaghetti cooked	1 cup	183	tr	tr
whole wheat cooked	1 cup (4.9 oz)	174	tr	tr
Bella Via Fettucini cooked	⅝ cup	200	0	0
Bella Via Penne cooked	⅝ cup	200	0	0
Classico Gnocchi Di Toscana	1 cup (2 oz)	210	0	1
Tree Of Life Tomato Basil as prep	⅝ cup (4.9 oz)	200	0	1
PASTA DINNERS				
lasagna	1 piece (2.5 in x 2.5 in)	374	11	21
manicotti	¾ cup (6.4 oz)	273	6	12
rigatoni w/ sausage sauce	¾ cup	260	4	12
spaghetti w/ meatballs & cheese	1 cup	407	6	19
Banquet Family Entree Macaroni & Beef	1 serv (8 oz)	230	3	7
Banquet Family Entree Macaroni & Cheese	1 serv (8 oz)	300	5	10
Chef Boyardee ABC's & 1,2,3's w/ Mini Meatballs	7.5 oz	260	4	11
Chef Boyardee Beef Ravioli	7.5 oz	190	2	4
Chef Boyardee Beefaroni	7.5 oz	220	1	7
Healthy Choice Cheese Ravioli Parmigiana	1 meal (9 oz)	250	2	4
Healthy Choice Chicken Fettucini Alfredo	1 meal (8.5 oz)	250	1	3

FOOD	PORTION	CALS.	SAT. FAT	TOTAL FAT
Healthy Choice Spaghetti Bolognese	1 meal (10 oz)	260	1	3
Healthy Choice Zucchini Lasagna	1 meal (14 oz)	330	1	2
Kid's Kitchen Spaghetti Rings & Franks	1 cup (7.5 oz)	230	3	6
Pasta Favorites Italian Sausage & Peppers	1 pkg (10.5 oz)	340	4	13
Pasta Favorites Pasta Primavera	1 pkg (10.5 oz)	320	6	14
Progresso Cheese Ravioli	1 cup (9.1 oz)	220	1	2
Weight Watchers Penne Pasta With Sun-Dried Tomatoes	1 pkg (10 oz)	290	3	9
Weight Watchers Spaghetti With Meat Sauce	1 pkg (10 oz)	250	2	6
Weight Watchers Tuna Noodle Casserole	1 pkg (9.5 oz)	240	3	7
PASTA FRESH				
Contadina Angel's Hair	1¼ cup (2.8 oz)	240	1	3
Contadina Light Ravioli Cheese	1 cup (3.1 oz)	240	2	5
Contadina Ravioli Cheese	1 cup (3.1 oz)	280	6	12
Di Giorno Fettuccine Spinach	2.5 oz	190	0	2
Di Giorno Ravioli With Italian Sausage	¾ cup (3.6 oz)	340	5	12
Di Giorno Tortellini With Chicken And Herbs	1 cup (3.2 oz)	260	3	5
PASTA SALAD				
elbow macaroni salad	1 cup	160	2	5
pasta salad w/ vegetables	1 cup	140	3	4
Kraft Pasta Salad Classic Ranch With Bacon	¾ cup (4.7 oz)	360	4	23
Kraft Pasta Salad Light Italian	¾ cup (5 oz)	190	1	2
PATE				
goose liver smoked	1 oz	131	—	12
Sells Liver	2.08 oz	190	—	16
PEACH				
fresh	1	37	tr	tr
Del Monte Halves Cling In Heavy Syrup	½ cup (4.5 oz)	100	0	0
Del Monte Halves Cling Lite	½ cup (4.4 oz)	60	0	0

FOOD	PORTION	CALS.	SAT. FAT	TOTAL FAT
Del Monte Sun Dried	⅓ cup (1.4 oz)	90	0	0
S&W Sliced Clingstone Diet	½ cup	30	0	0
S&W Whole Yellow Cling Spiced In Heavy Syrup	½ cup	90	0	0
Snapple Dixie Peach Juice	10 fl oz	140	0	0
PEANUT BUTTER				
Crazy Richard's Natural Creamy	2 tbsp (1.1 oz)	190	2	16
Estee Chunky Sodium Free	2 tbsp (1 oz)	190	3	15
Jif Simply Creamy	2 tbsp (1.1 oz)	190	3	16
Peter Pan Creamy	2 tbsp	190	2	16
Skippy Creamy w/ 2 slices white bread	1 sandwich	340	3	19
Skippy Reduced Fat Creamy	2 tbsp	190	3	12
Smucker's Goober Grape	2 tbsp	180	2	10
Smucker's Natural	2 tbsp	200	3	16
Tree Of Life Creamy Organic	2 tbsp (1 oz)	190	4	16
PEANUTS				
chocolate coated	10 (1.4 oz)	208	6	13
Little Debbie Salted	1 pkg (1.2 oz)	230	3	21
Planters Cocktail Lightly Salted Oil Roasted	1 oz	170	2	15
Planters Heat Hot Spicy Oil Roasted	1 pkg (1.7 oz)	290	4	25
Planters Honey Roasted	1 oz	160	2	13
Planters Reduced Fat Honey Roasted	⅓ cup (1 oz)	130	1	7
PEAR				
asian	1 (4.3 oz)	51	tr	tr
dried halves	5	230	0	tr
fresh	1	98	tr	1
Del Monte Halves Fruit Naturals	½ cup (4.4 oz)	60	0	0
Del Monte Halves In Heavy Syrup	½ cup (4.5 oz)	100	0	0
Del Monte Halves Lite	½ cup (4.4 oz)	60	0	0
Del Monte Snack Cups Diced Lite	1 serv (4.5 oz)	60	0	0
Kern's Nectar	6 fl oz	120	0	0
PEAS				
fresh green cooked	½ cup	67	tr	tr
fresh green raw	½ cup	58	tr	tr

FOOD	PORTION	CALS.	SAT. FAT	TOTAL FAT
pea & potato curry	1 serv (7 oz)	284	—	22
sugar snap cooked	½ cup	34	tr	tr
sugar snap raw	½ cup	30	tr	tr
Birds Eye In Butter Sauce	½ cup	80	1	2
Chun King Snow Pea Pods frzn	½ pkg (3 oz)	35	0	2
S&W Petit Pois	½ cup	70	0	0
PECANS				
Planters Halves	1 oz	190	2	20
Planters Honey Roasted	1 oz	180	2	16
PECTIN				
Slim Set Powder	1 tbsp	3	0	0
PEPPER				
Ac'cent Lemon	½ tsp	0	0	0
Watkins Cracked Black	¼ tbsp (0.5 g)	0	0	0
Watkins Red Pepper Flakes	¼ tsp (0.5 oz)	0	0	0
PEPPERS				
chili green hot raw chopped	¼ cup	15	tr	tr
chili red raw chopped	¼ cup	15	tr	tr
green raw	½ (1.3 oz)	10	0	tr
red raw	½ (1.3 oz)	10	0	tr
yellow raw	10 strips	14	—	tr
Del Monte Hot Chili	4 (1 oz)	10	0	0
Del Monte Jalapeno Nacho Pickled Sliced	2 tbsp (1 oz)	5	0	0
Hebrew National Hot Cherry	⅓ pepper (1 oz)	11	0	0
Old El Paso Green Chilies Chopped	2 tbsp (1 oz)	5	0	0
Progresso Pepper Salad (drained)	2 tbsp (0.9 oz)	25	0	2
Progresso Roasted	½ piece (1 oz)	10	0	0
Trappey Serano	7 peppers (1 oz)	7	tr	tr
PERCH				
cooked	3 oz	99	tr	1
Van De Kamp's Battered Fillets	2 (4 oz)	300	3	20
PERSIMMONS				
fresh	1	118	0	tr
Sonoma Dried	6–8 pieces (1.4 oz)	140	0	0
PICKLES				
Del Monte Dill Halves	¼ pickle (1 oz)	5	0	0
Del Monte Dill Hamburger Chips	5 pieces (1 oz)	5	0	0

FOOD	PORTION	CALS.	SAT. FAT	TOTAL FAT
Del Monte Dill Sweet Gherkin	2 pickles (1 oz)	40	0	0
Hebrew National Half Sour	½ pickle (1 oz)	4	0	0
Hebrew National Kosher	⅓ pickle (1 oz)	4	0	0
McIlhenny Hot N' Sweet	4 (1 oz)	42	tr	tr
Vlasic Bread & Butter Chips	1 oz	30	0	0
Vlasic Hot & Spicy Garden Mix	1 oz	4	0	0
PIE				
apple fried	1 (6.4 oz)	404	3	21
banana cream	⅛ of 9 in pie (5.2 oz)	398	6	20
blueberry	⅛ of 9 in pie (5.2 oz)	360	4	18
coconut creme	⅛ of 9 in pie (4.7 oz)	396	8	21
coconut custard	⅙ of 8 in pie (3.6 oz)	271	6	14
lemon meringue	⅛ of 9 in pie (4.5 oz)	362	4	16
pecan	⅙ of 8 in pie (4 oz)	452	4	21
pumpkin	⅙ of 8 in pie (3.8 oz)	229	2	10
Lance Pecan Snack	1 (38 g)	350	3	15
Little Debbie Raisin Creme Snack	1 pkg (1.2 oz)	140	1	5
Tastykake Cherry Snack	1 pkg (113 g)	300	2	10
Tastykake Lemon Lime Snack	1 pkg (113 g)	320	3	13
PIEROGI				
Empire Potato Cheese	3 (4.6 oz)	260	3	6
Golden Potato Onion	3 (4 oz)	210	2	6
PIGEON PEAS				
dried cooked	½ cup	102	tr	tr
PIG'S EARS AND FEET				
Hormel Pickled Feet	2 oz	80	2	6
PIKE				
cooked	3 oz	96	tr	1
PIMIENTOS				
canned	1 tbsp	3	tr	tr
PINE NUTS				
Progresso Pignoli	1 jar (1 oz)	170	1	13

FOOD	PORTION	CALS.	SAT. FAT	TOTAL FAT
PINEAPPLE				
fresh diced	1 cup	77	tr	tr
fresh slice	1 slice	42	tr	tr
Del Monte Chunks In Its Own Juice	½ cup (4.4 oz)	70	0	0
Del Monte Juice	8 fl oz	110	0	0
Empress Crushed	4 oz	70	0	0
PINK BEANS				
Goya Spanish Style	7.5 oz	140	0	tr
PINTO BEANS				
Allen Canned	½ cup (4.5 oz)	110	0	1
Eden Organic	½ cup (4.4 oz)	90	0	1
PISTACHIOS				
Planters Munch'N Go Singles Shelled Dry Roasted	1 pkg (2 oz)	330	4	29
Planters Uncolored Dry Roasted	½ cup	160	2	14
PIZZA				
cheese	⅛ of 12 in pie	140	2	3
cheese deep dish individual	1 (5.5 oz)	460	9	24
cheese meat & vegetables	⅛ of 12 in pie	184	2	5
pepperoni	⅛ of 12 in pie	181	2	7
Boboli Shell + Sauce	⅛ lg shell (2.6 oz)	170	1	3
Celeste Italian Bread Deluxe	1 (5.1 oz)	290	3	11
Croissant Pocket Stuffed Sandwich Pepperoni Pizza	1 piece (4.5 oz)	350	5	15
Empire Bagel	1 (2 oz)	150	3	5
Empire English Muffin	1 (2 oz)	130	3	5
Healthy Choice French Bread Pepperoni	1 (6 oz)	360	4	9
Kid Cuisine Hamburger	1 (8.30 oz)	400	4	11
Lean Pockets Stuffed Sandwich Pizza Deluxe	1 (4.5 oz)	270	3	8
Old El Paso Pizza Burrito Cheese	1 (3.5 oz)	320	4	9
Special Delivery Organic	⅓ pizza (5.3 oz)	320	5	9
Stouffer's French Bread Garden Vegetable	1 piece (5.8 oz)	340	4	12
Tombstone 12 in Canadian Bacon	⅕ pie (5.5 oz)	360	7	15
Tombstone 12 in Extra Cheese	⅕ pie (5.1 oz)	370	9	17

FOOD	PORTION	CALS.	SAT. FAT	TOTAL FAT
Tombstone 12 in Special Order Four Meat	⅙ pie (4.7 oz)	350	8	18
Tombstone For One 1/2 Less Fat Cheese	1 pie (6.5 oz)	360	5	10
Tombstone For One 1/2 Less Fat Vegetable	1 pie (7.2 oz)	360	4	10
Weight Watchers Deluxe Combo	1 (6.57 oz)	380	4	11
PLANTAINS				
fried	½ cup	214	—	7
sliced cooked	½ cup	89	0	tr
Chifles Plantain Chips	1 pkg (2 oz)	170	2	11
PLUMS				
fresh	1	36	tr	tr
S&W Whole Purple Fancy Unpeeled In Extra Heavy Syrup	½ cup	135	0	0
S&W Whole Unpeeled Diet	½ cup	52	0	0
POLENTA				
Aurora Polenta	½ cup (5 oz)	110	0	0
POLLACK				
baked	3 oz	100	tr	1
POMEGRANATES				
pomegranate	1	104	0	tr
POMPANO				
florida cooked	3 oz	179	4	10
POPCORN				
air-popped	1 cup (0.3 oz)	31	tr	tr
caramel coated	1 cup (1.2 oz)	152	1	5
carmel coated w/ peanuts	⅔ cup (1 oz)	114	tr	2
cheese	1 cup (0.4 oz)	58	1	4
oil popped	1 cup (0.4 oz)	55	1	3
General Mills Popcorn Bars Caramel	1 (0.6 oz)	70	1	1
Jiffy Pop Bag Butter	3 cups	90	1	5
Jiffy Pop Bag Lite	3 cups	70	tr	3
Lance Plain	1 pkg (25 g)	140	2	9
Louise's Fat-Free Apple Cinnamon	1 oz	100	0	0
Newman's Own Oldstyle Picture Show Microwave Natural Butter	3 cups	150	2	8

FOOD	PORTION	CALS.	SAT. FAT	TOTAL FAT
Orville Redenbacher's Microwave Gourmet Butter	3 cups	100	1	6
Orville Redenbacher's Microwave Gourmet Light	3 cups	70	1	3
Pop Secret Light Butter Flavor Singles	6 cups	140	1	6
Weight Watchers White Cheddar Cheese	1 pkg (0.66 oz)	90	1	4
POPCORN CAKES				
Mother's Butter Flavor	1 (0.3 oz)	35	0	0
Quaker Caramel	1 (0.5 oz)	50	0	0
Quaker White Cheddar	1 (0.4 oz)	40	0	0
POPOVER				
popover	1 (1.4 oz)	87	1	3
PORK				
chop loin bone-in lean & fat roasted	3 oz	199	4	11
center loin roasted	3 oz	259	7	18
ham fresh rump half lean & fat roasted	3 oz	233	—	23
chop rib bone-in lean & fat roasted	3 oz	217	5	13
rib chop lean & fat panfried	1 chop (2.9 oz)	343	—	29
spareribs braised	3 oz	338	10	26
tenderloin lean only roasted	3 oz	141	1	4
PORK DISHES				
pork roast	2 oz	70	1	3
Jimmy Dean BBQ Pork Rib Sandwich	1 (5.4 oz)	440	7	23
POT PIE				
Award Brand Beef	1 (7 oz)	350	8	18
Banquet Family Entree Chicken Pie	1 serv (8 oz)	450	12	30
Banquet Macaroni & Cheese	1 pkg (6.5 oz)	200	2	3
Banquet Vegetable & Cheese	1 (7 oz)	390	8	18
Empire Turkey	1 (8.1 oz)	470	5	23
POTATO				
au gratin w/ cheese	½ cup	178	4	10
baked topped w/ cheese sauce	1	475	11	29

FOOD	PORTION	CALS.	SAT. FAT	TOTAL FAT
baked topped w/ cheese sauce & broccoli	1	402	9	14
baked topped w/ cheese sauce & chili	1	481	13	22
baked topped w/ sour cream & chives	1	394	10	22
baked w/ skin	1 (6.5 oz)	220	tr	tr
boiled	½ cup	68	tr	tr
french fried	1 reg	235	4	12
hash brown	½ cup	163	4	11
instant mashed flakes as prep w/ whole milk & butter	½ cup	118	4	6
mashed	⅔ cup	132	tr	1
microwaved	1 (7 oz)	212	tr	tr
mustard potato salad	½ cup	120	0	6
potato salad	½ cup	179	2	10
Del Monte New Whole	⅔ cup (5.5 oz)	60	0	0
Hormel Scalloped & Ham	1 can (7.5 oz)	260	5	16
Kineret Crinkle Cut frzn	18 pieces (3 oz)	120	1	4
Kineret Kugel	1 piece (2.5 oz)	150	2	10
Kineret Latkes	1 (1.5 oz)	90	—	5
Ore Ida Cottage Fries	14 pieces (3 oz)	130	1	4
Ore Ida Microwave Tater Tots	1 pkg (3.75 oz)	190	3	10
Ore Ida Toaster Hash Browns	2 patties (3.5 oz)	190	2	12
Yukon Gold Fresh	1 (5.3 oz)	110	0	0
PRETZELS				
chocolate covered	1 (0.4 oz)	50	1	2
whole wheat	2 med (2 oz)	205	tr	2
Barrel O' Fun Sticks	1 oz	110	0	1
Estee Dutch Unsalted	2 (1.1 oz)	130	0	1
Formagg Pretzel Nuts	1 oz	120	1	4
Manischewitz Bagel Pretzels Original	4 (1 oz)	110	0	0
Mr. Phipps Chips Original	16 (1 oz)	120	0	3
Mr. Phipps Chips Original Fat Free	16 (1 oz)	100	0	0
Planters Twists	1 oz	100	0	1
Quinlan Hard Sourdough	1 oz	110	1	2
Snyder's Logs	1 oz	310	0	0

FOOD	PORTION	CALS.	SAT. FAT	TOTAL FAT
PRUNE JUICE				
Del Monte Juice	8 fl oz	170	0	0
S&W Unsweetened	6 oz	120	0	0
PRUNES				
in heavy syrup	1 cup	245	tr	tr
Del Monte Pitted	¼ cup (1.4 oz)	120	0	0
Sunsweet Orange Essence Pitted Prunes	6 (1.4 oz)	100	0	0
PUDDING				
bread pudding	½ cup (4.4 oz)	212	3	7
chocolate	½ cup (5.5 oz)	206	2	4
rice pudding	1 serv (3 oz)	110	—	4
rice w/ raisins	½ cup	246	3	6
tapioca	½ cup (5.3 oz)	189	—	7
vanilla	½ cup (4.3 oz)	130	3	4
Del Monte Snack Cups Butterscotch	1 serv (4 oz)	140	1	4
Del Monte Snack Cups Chocolate	1 serv (4 oz)	160	1	4
Del Monte Snack Cups Lite Chocolate	1 serv (4 oz)	100	0	1
Hunt's Snack Pack Banana	1 (4 oz)	158	2	6
Hunt's Snack Pack Fat Free Chocolate	1 (4 oz)	96	0	tr
Hunt's Snack Pack Fat Free Tapioca	1 (4 oz)	95	0	tr
Hunt's Snack Pack Fat Free Vanilla	1 (4 oz)	93	0	tr
Imagine Foods Lemon Dream	1 (4 oz)	120	0	0
Swiss Miss Light Vanilla Chocolate Parfait	4 oz	100	tr	1
PUMPKIN				
salted & roasted seeds	1 oz	148	2	12
QUICHE				
lorraine	⅛ of 8 in pie	600	23	48
mushroom	1 slice (3 oz)	256	—	18
QUINOA				
Arrowhead Quinoa	¼ cup (1.4 oz)	140	0	2
RABBIT				
domestic w/o bone roasted	3 oz	167	2	7

FOOD	PORTION	CALS.	SAT. FAT	TOTAL FAT
RADICCHIO				
raw shredded	½ cup	5	0	tr
RADISHES				
daikon raw sliced	½ cup	8	tr	tr
red raw	10	7	tr	tr
white icicle raw sliced	½ cup	7	tr	tr
RAISINS				
chocolate coated	10 (0.4 oz)	39	1	2
golden seedless	¼ cup	109	0	tr
Del Monte Snack Size	1 box (1.5 oz)	140	0	0
Del Monte Yogurt Raisins Vanilla	1 pkg (0.9 oz)	110	3	3
Tree Of Life Organic	¼ cup (1.4 oz)	130	0	0
RASPBERRIES				
fresh	½ cup	31	0	0
Big Valley Raspberries frzn	⅔ cup (4.9 oz)	80	0	0
Crystal Geyser Juice Squeeze Mountain Raspberry	1 bottle (12 fl oz)	135	0	0
RED BEANS				
Allen Canned	½ cup (4.5 oz)	160	0	1
Mahatma Red Beans & Rice	1 cup	190	0	1
RELISH				
cranberry orange	¼ cup	123	0	tr
Del Monte Hamburger	1 tbsp (0.5 oz)	20	0	0
Old El Paso Jalapeno	1 tbsp (0.5 oz)	5	0	0
Vlasic Hot Piccalilli	1 oz	35	0	0
Vlasic Sweet	1 oz	30	0	0
RHUBARB				
frzn as prep w/ sugar	½ cup	139	0	tr
RICE				
brown cooked	½ cup	109	tr	tr
glutinous cooked	½ cup	116	tr	tr
pilaf	½ cup	84	1	3
risotto	6.6 oz	426	—	18
spanish	¾ cup	363	10	27
Arrowhead Basmati Brown	¼ cup (1.5 oz)	150	0	1
Arrowhead Quick Regular	⅓ cup (1.5 oz)	150	0	1
Casbah Jambalaya	1 pkg (1.4 oz)	130	0	0
Casbah Thai Yum	1 pkg (1.7 oz)	180	0	3

FOOD	PORTION	CALS.	SAT. FAT	TOTAL FAT
Chun King Fried Rice	1 pkg (8 oz)	290	2	6
Lipton Golden Saute Chicken	1 cup (2.2 oz)	240	2	5
Lipton Rice & Sauce Cajun as prep	½ cup (2.2 oz)	230	0	1
Mahatma Yellow Rice Mix	1 cup	190	0	0
Near East Curry Rice as prep	1 cup	220	1	4
Near East Long Grain & Wild as prep	1 cup	220	1	5
Success Classic Chicken	½ cup	150	0	1
Superfino Arborio Rice	½ cup	100	0	0
Uncle Ben Boil-In-Bag	1 serv (0.9 oz)	94	0	tr
Uncle Ben Converted	1 serv (1.2 oz)	123	0	tr
RICE CAKES				
Ka-Me Mini Plain	16 pieces (1 oz)	120	0	2
Lundberg Organic Unsalted	1	60	0	1
Mother's Mini Caramel	5 (0.5 oz)	50	0	0
Pritikin Multigrain	1 (0.3 oz)	35	0	0
Quaker Apple Cinnamon	1 (0.5 oz)	50	0	0
Quaker Mini White Cheddar	6 (0.5 oz)	50	0	0
Tree Of Life Fat Free Mini Jalapeno	15	60	0	0
ROE				
fresh baked	1 oz	58	1	2
ROLL				
cheese	1 (2.3 oz)	238	4	12
egg	1 (2½ in)	107	1	2
hard	1 (3½ in)	167	tr	2
kaiser	1 (3½ in)	167	tr	2
rye	1 (1 oz)	81	tr	1
submarine	1 (4.7 oz)	155	tr	2
Alvarado St. Bakery Hot Dog Buns	1 (2.2 oz)	140	0	2
Arnold Dinner Plain	1 (0.7 oz)	50	0	1
Bread Du Jour Sourdough	1 (2.2 oz)	140	0	2
Dicarlo's French	1 (1 oz)	70	0	1
Home Pride Hamburger Potato Bun	1 (1.9 oz)	130	0	2
Pepperidge Farm Brown 'N Serve French	½ roll	180	1	2
Pepperidge Farm Finger Poppy Seed	1	50	0	2

FOOD	PORTION	CALS.	SAT. FAT	TOTAL FAT
Pepperidge Farm Frankfurter Dijon	1	160	1	5
Pillsbury Crescent refrigerated	1	100	1	6
Roman Meal Sandwich	1 (2.7 oz)	181	tr	3
Weight Watchers Glazed Cinnamon Rolls	1 (2.1 oz)	200	2	5
Wonder Hamburger Light	1 (1.5 oz)	80	0	2
Wonder Hot Dog Light	1 (1.5 oz)	80	0	2
ROUGHY				
orange baked	3 oz	75	tr	1
RUTABAGA				
cooked mashed	½ cup	41	tr	tr
SABLEFISH				
smoked	1 oz	72	1	6
SALAD				
chef w/o dressing	1½ cups	386	13	28
tossed w/o dressing w/ chicken	1½ cups	105	tr	2
tossed w/o dressing w/ pasta & seafood	1½ cups (14.6 oz)	380	3	21
waldorf	½ cup	79	2	6
Dole Caesar Salad	⅓ pkg (3.5 oz)	170	2	14
Dole Salad-In-A-Minute Spinach	3.5 oz	180	2	9
Fresh Express Garden Salad	1½ cups (3 oz)	20	0	0
Fresh Express Oriental Salad	1½ cups (3 oz)	120	1	8
SALAD DRESSING				
Kraft Buttermilk Ranch	2 tbsp (1 oz)	150	3	16
Kraft Catalina With Honey	2 tbsp (1.2 oz)	140	2	12
Kraft Free French	2 tbsp (1.2 oz)	50	0	0
Kraft Free Peppercorn Ranch	2 tbsp (1.2 oz)	50	0	0
Kraft Oil-Free Italian	2 tbsp (1.1 oz)	5	0	0
Kraft Russian	2 tbsp (1.2 oz)	130	2	10
Marzetti Fat Free Slaw	2 tbsp	45	0	0
Marzetti Light Red Wine Vinegar & Oil	2 tbsp	20	0	1
Marzetti Light Slaw	2 tbsp	60	1	7
Marzetti Old Fashioned Poppyseed	2 tbsp	140	2	11
Newman's Own Olive Oil & Vinegar	1 tbsp (0.5 fl oz)	80	1	9
Pritikin Dijon Balsamic Vinaigrette	2 tbsp (1 oz)	3	0	0
Seven Seas Free Red Wine Vinegar	2 tbsp (1.1 oz)	15	0	0

FOOD	PORTION	CALS.	SAT. FAT	TOTAL FAT
Seven Seas Red Wine Vinegar & Oil	2 tbsp (1.1 oz)	110	2	11
W.J. Clark Lime Cilantro Vinaigrette	1 tbsp	73	1	8
Walden Farms Fat Free Raspberry Vinaigrette	2 tbsp (1 oz)	20	0	0
Weight Watchers Fat Free Caesar	2 tbsp	10	0	0
Weight Watchers Fat Free Honey Dijon	2 tbsp	45	0	0
Wishbone Chunky Blue Cheese	2 tbsp (1 oz)	170	3	17
Wishbone Creamy Italian	2 tbsp (1 oz)	100	2	10
Wishbone Fat Free Chunky Blue Cheese	2 tbsp (1 oz)	35	0	0
Wishbone Fat Free Italian	2 tbsp (1 oz)	15	0	0
SALMON				
pink baked	3 oz	127	1	4
salmon cake	1 (3 oz)	241	7	15
Bumble Bee Pink canned	3.5 oz	160	2	8
Bumble Bee Red canned	3.5 oz	180	2	10
Nathan's Nova	2 oz	80	1	3
SALSA				
Chi-Chi's Hot	2 tbsp (1 oz)	10	0	0
Del Monte Verde	2 tbsp (1.1 oz)	10	0	0
Guiltless Gourmet Picante Hot	1 oz	6	0	0
Heluva Good Cheese Cheese & Salsa	2 tbsp (1.1 oz)	80	5	6
Hunt's Mild	2 tbsp (1.1 oz)	27	0	tr
Louise's Fat Free BBQ Black Bean	1 oz	10	0	0
Newman's Own Bandito Medium	1 tbsp (0.7 oz)	6	0	tr
Old El Paso Homestyle	2 tbsp (1 oz)	5	0	0
Rosarita Taco Salsa Chunky Medium	3 tbsp (1.5 oz)	25	0	tr
SALT/SEASONED SALT				
salt	1 tsp (6 g)	0	0	0
Cardia Salt Alternative	1 pkg (0.6 g)	0	0	0
Hain Sea Salt	1 tsp	0	0	0
Morton Lite	1 tsp	tr	0	0
Morton Seasoned	1 tsp	4	0	tr

FOOD	PORTION	CALS.	SAT. FAT	TOTAL FAT
SAPODILLA				
fresh	1	140	—	2
SARDINES				
Del Monte In Tomato Sauce	1 fish (1.4 oz)	50	1	3
Empress Skinless & Boneless Olive Oil	1 can (3.8 oz)	420	—	38
Port Clyde In Mustard Sauce	1 can (3.75 oz)	150	2	9
Underwood With Tabasco Pepper Sauce drained	3 oz	220	—	16
Viking's Delight Brisling In Olive Oil drained	1 can (3.75 oz)	260	—	20
SAUCE				
Best Foods Tartar	1 tbsp (0.5 oz)	70	1	8
Casa Fiesta Taco Mild	1 oz	9	—	tr
Del Monte Cocktail	¼ cup (2.7 oz)	100	0	0
Gebhardt Enchilada Sauce	3 tbsp (1.5 oz)	25	1	1
Heinz Worcestershire	1 tbsp	6	0	0
House Of Tsang Hoisin	1 tsp (6 g)	15	0	0
Ka-Me Duck Sauce	2 tbsp (1 oz)	80	0	0
Ka-Me Tamari	1 tbsp (0.5 fl oz)	10	0	1
Kraft Sweet'n Sour	2 tbsp (1.3 oz)	80	0	1
Lea & Perrins Steak	1 oz	40	—	tr
McIlhenny Tabasco	1 tsp	1	tr	tr
Progresso Alfredo	½ cup (4.4 oz)	310	15	27
SAUERKRAUT				
S&W Canned	½ cup	25	0	0
S&W Juice	4 oz	14	0	0
SAUSAGE				
bratwurst pork cooked	1 link (3 oz)	256	8	22
link	1 (0.5 oz)	48	1	4
sausage roll	1 (2.3 oz)	311	—	24
Aidells Andouille Cajun Cooked	1 (3.5 oz)	220	8	17
Healthy Choice Low Fat Smoked	2 oz	70	1	2
Hillshire Flavorseal Kielbasa Polska Lite	2 oz	130	—	11
Hormel Vienna	2 oz	140	4	13
Jimmy Dean Pattie Pre-Cooked	1 (1.9 oz)	230	8	22
Jones Italian	1	160	—	14

FOOD	PORTION	CALS.	SAT. FAT	TOTAL FAT
Jones Scrapple	1 slice (1.5 oz)	90	—	6
Little Sizzlers Brown & Serve	3 links (2.1 oz)	190	8	22
Louis Rich Turkey	2.5 oz	110	3	6
Oscar Mayer Smokies Cheese	1 (1.5 oz)	130	4	12
Perdue Breakfast Links Turkey Cooked	2 links (2 oz)	100	2	6
Shofar Knockwurst Beef	1 (3 oz)	260	9	23
SAUSAGE SUBSTITUTES				
Morningstar Farms Breakfast Links	2 (45 g)	90	—	5
White Wave Meatless Healthy Links	2 (1.6 oz)	140	2	10
SCALLOP				
breaded & fried	2 lg	67	1	3
SCONE				
plain	1 (1.75 oz)	181	—	7
raisin	1 (1.75 oz)	158	—	5
SEAWEED				
Eden Agar Agar Flakes	1 tbsp (2.5 oz)	10	0	0
Eden Kombu	3.5 in piece (3.3 g)	10	0	0
Eden Nori	1 sheet (2.5 g)	10	0	0
Eden Wakame	½ cup (0.3 oz)	25	0	0
Maine Coast Dulse	⅓ cup (7 g)	18	0	0
Maine Coast Kelp	⅓ cup (7 g)	17	0	0
SESAME				
sesame crunch candy	10 pieces (0.6 oz)	90	1	6
Joyva Tahini	2 tbsp (1 oz)	200	3	18
Planters Nut Mix	1 oz	150	2	12
SHAD				
baked	3 oz	214	—	15
roe baked w/ butter & lemon	3.5 oz	126	—	3
SHARK				
batter-dipped & fried	3 oz	194	3	12
SHELLFISH SUBSTITUTES				
surimi	1 oz	28	—	tr
Louis Kemp Crab Delights Chunk Style	2 oz	54	—	tr

FOOD	PORTION	CALS.	SAT. FAT	TOTAL FAT
SHERBET				
Hood Orange	½ cup (3.1 oz)	120	1	1
Sealtest Rainbow Orange Red Raspberry Lime	½ cup (3 oz)	130	1	1
SHRIMP				
breaded & fried	6 to 8 (6 oz)	454	5	25
cooked	4 large	22	tr	tr
Van De Kamp's Breaded Butterfly	7 (4 oz)	280	3	14
Van De Kamp's Breaded Popcorn	20 (4 oz)	270	2	13
SMELT				
cooked	3 oz	106	tr	3
SNACKS				
Cheetos Curls	15 pieces (1 oz)	150	—	9
Cheetos Light	38 pieces (1 oz)	140	—	6
Chex Snack Mix Barbeque	½ cup (1.1 oz)	130	1	5
Combos Cheddar Cheese Pretzel	1 pkg (1.8 oz)	240	2	9
Combos Peanut Butter Cracker	1 oz	140	2	8
Cornnuts Original	1 pkg (2 oz)	260	2	8
Energy Food Factory Poprice Cheddar Cheese	½ oz	60	—	3
Energy Food Factory Poprice Lite	½ oz	50	—	2
Handi-Snacks Peanut Butter'n Crackers	1 pkg (1.1 oz)	180	3	12
Planters Cheez Balls	1 oz	150	2	10
Weight Watchers Pizza Curls	1 pkg (0.5 oz)	60	0	2
SNAIL				
cooked	3 oz	233	tr	1
SNAPPER				
cooked	3 oz	109	tr	1
SODA				
7 Up Diet	1 oz	tr	0	0
7 Up Original	1 oz	12	0	0
Barrelhead Root Beer	8 fl oz	110	0	0
Canada Dry Club	8 fl oz	0	0	0
Canada Dry Diet Tonic Water	8 fl oz	0	0	0
Canada Dry Seltzer Lemon Lime	8 fl oz	0	0	0

FOOD	PORTION	CALS.	SAT. FAT	TOTAL FAT
Clearly Canadian Country Raspberry	8 fl oz	80	0	0
Coca-Cola Cherry	8 fl oz	104	0	0
Coca-Cola Classic	8 fl oz	97	0	0
Coca-Cola Diet	8 fl oz	1	0	0
Cott Grape	8 fl oz	130	0	0
Crush Orange	8 fl oz	140	0	0
Dr Pepper Diet	8 oz	tr	0	0
Dr Pepper Original	8 oz	104	0	0
Fresca Soda	8 fl oz	3	0	0
Hires Cream	8 fl oz	130	0	0
Hires Cream Soda Diet	8 fl oz	0	0	0
Lucozade Soda	7 oz	136	0	0
Manischewitz Seltzer No Salt Added No Calories	8 fl oz	0	0	0
Mello Yellow Diet	8 fl oz	4	0	0
Mountain Dew Diet	8 fl oz	2	0	0
Mountain Dew Soda	8 fl oz	118	0	0
Mr. PiBB Diet	8 fl oz	1	0	0
Nehi Fruit Punch	8 fl oz	120	0	0
Nehi Quinine Water	8 fl oz	90	0	0
Orangina Sparkling Citrus	6 fl oz	80	0	0
Pepsi Diet	8 fl oz	1	0	0
Pepsi Regular	8 fl oz	105	0	0
Schweppes Bitter Lemon	8 fl oz	110	0	0
Slice Diet Lemon Lime	8 fl oz	5	0	0
Slice Lemon Lime	8 fl oz	100	0	0
Sprite Diet	8 fl oz	3	0	0
Sprite Soda	8 fl oz	100	0	0
Welch's Sparkling Grape	12 oz	180	0	0
Yoo-Hoo Original	9 fl oz	150	tr	tr
SOLE				
cooked	1 fillet (4.5 oz)	148	tr	2
Van De Kamp's Lightly Breaded Fillets	1 (4 oz)	220	2	11
SOUFFLE				
cheese	3.5 oz	253	—	20

FOOD	PORTION	CALS.	SAT. FAT	TOTAL FAT
SOUP				
beef stew soup	1 cup (8.8 oz)	221	2	5
black bean turtle soup	1 cup	241	tr	1
corn & cheese chowder	¾ cup	215	7	12
gazpacho	1 cup	46	0	tr
greek lemon soup	¾ cup	63	1	2
hot & sour	1 serv (14 oz)	173	2	8
pasta e fagioll	1 cup (8.8 oz)	194	1	5
Campbell Asparagus Cream Of as prep	8 oz	80	—	4
Campbell Celery Cream Of as prep	8 oz	100	—	7
Campbell Cheddar Cheese as prep	8 oz	110	—	6
Campbell Chicken & Pasta With Garden Vegetables	1 cup (8.4 oz)	90	0	1
Campbell Consomme as prep	8 oz	25	—	0
Campbell Mushroom Cream Of as prep	8 oz	100	—	7
Campbell Tomato as prep	8 oz	90	—	2
Campbell Vegetarian Vegetable as prep	8 oz	80	—	2
Casbah Vegetarian Chili	1 pkg (1.8 oz)	170	0	2
College Inn Beef Broth	½ can (7 oz)	16	0	0
College Inn Chicken Broth Lower Salt	½ can (7 oz)	20	1	2
Cup-A-Soup Chicken Noodle as prep	1 pkg	50	1	1
Gold's Borscht	8 oz	100	0	0
Gold's Borscht Lo-Cal	8 oz	20	0	tr
Gold's Schav	8 oz	25	0	0
Goodman's Matzo Ball & Soup	1 cup	40	0	1
Hain Mushroom Barley	9.5 fl oz	100	—	2
Hain Turkey Rice	9.5 fl oz	100	—	3
Hain Vegetable Broth	9.5 fl oz	45	0	0
Health Valley Green Split Pea	7.5 oz	180	—	tr
Health Valley Lentil	7.5 oz	220	—	4
Healthy Choice Vegetable Beef	1 cup (8.8 oz)	130	tr	1
Hormel Bean & Ham	1 cup (7.5 oz)	190	2	4
Kojel Tomato Instant	1 serv (6 fl oz)	50	0	0

FOOD	PORTION	CALS.	SAT. FAT	TOTAL FAT
Lipton Recipe Secrets Golden Onion	2 tbsp	60	0	2
Lipton Soup Secrets Giggle Noodle	1 serv	80	1	2
Maruchan Ramen Beef	½ pkg (1.5 oz)	190	—	9
Progresso Chickarina	1 cup (8.3 oz)	120	2	5
Progresso Escarole In Chicken Broth	1 cup (8.1 oz)	25	0	1
Progresso Minestrone	1 can (10.5 fl oz)	170	1	4
Snow's Manhattan Clam Chowder as prep w/ water	7.5 fl oz	70	—	2
Snow's New England Clam Chowder as prep w/ milk	7.5 fl oz	140	—	6
Snow's New England Fish Chowder as prep w/ milk	7.5 fl oz	130	—	6
Swanson Natural Goodness Clear Chicken Broth	7.25 oz	20	—	1
Tabatchnick Cabbage	1 serv (7.5 oz)	60	0	0
Tabatchnick Spinach Cream Of	1 serv (7.5 oz)	90	2	4
Weight Watchers Chicken & Rice	1 can (10.5 oz)	110	0	2

SOUR CREAM

FOOD	PORTION	CALS.	SAT. FAT	TOTAL FAT
sour cream	1 tbsp	26	2	3
Breakstone Free	2 tbsp (1.1 oz)	35	0	0
Sealtest Light	2 tbsp (1.1 oz)	40	2	3

SOUR CREAM SUBSTITUTES

FOOD	PORTION	CALS.	SAT. FAT	TOTAL FAT
Tofutti Better Than Sour Cream Sour Supreme	1 oz	50	2	5

SOY

FOOD	PORTION	CALS.	SAT. FAT	TOTAL FAT
lecithin	1 tbsp	104	2	14
soya cheese	1.4 oz	128	—	11

SOY SAUCE

FOOD	PORTION	CALS.	SAT. FAT	TOTAL FAT
Eden Shoyu Organic	1 tbsp (0.5 oz)	15	0	0
House Of Tsang Light	1 tbsp (0.6 oz)	5	0	0
Tree Of Life Tamari Reduced Sodium	1 tbsp (0.5 oz)	20	0	0

SOYBEANS

FOOD	PORTION	CALS.	SAT. FAT	TOTAL FAT
green cooked	½ cup	127	1	6
roasted & toasted salted	1 oz	129	1	7
sprouts stir fried	1 cup	125	1	7

FOOD	PORTION	CALS.	SAT. FAT	TOTAL FAT
SPAGHETTI SAUCE				
bolognese	1 cup	195	—	15
Classico Ripe Olives & Mushrooms	4 fl oz	50	—	2
Contadina Alfredo	½ cup (4.2 fl oz)	400	21	38
Contadina Light Alfredo	½ cup (4.2 fl oz)	190	7	13
Contadina Pesto With Basil	¼ cup (2 oz)	310	5	30
Di Giorno Four Cheese	¼ cup (2.2 oz)	200	11	19
Di Giorno Light Reduced Fat Alfredo	¼ cup (2.4 oz)	170	6	10
Di Giorno Traditional Meat	½ cup (4.5 oz)	120	2	6
Eden Organic	½ cup (4.4 oz)	80	0	3
Hunt's Chunky Marinara	½ cup (4.4 oz)	60	tr	2
Mama Rizzo's Pepper Primavera Vegetable	½ cup (4.2 oz)	50	0	2
Muir Glen Organic Fat Free Tomato Basil	½ cup (4.3 oz)	50	0	0
Newman's Own Sockarooni	4 oz	70	—	2
Prego Mushroom	4 oz	130	—	5
Pritikin Chunky Garden	½ cup (4 oz)	50	0	1
Ragu Gardenstyle Chunky Garden Combination	½ cup (4.5 oz)	120	1	4
Tree Of Life Pasta Sauce Calabrese	½ cup (3.9 oz)	60	—	3
Weight Watchers Pasta Sauce With Mushrooms	½ cup	60	0	0
SPANISH FOOD				
burrito w/ beans	2 (7.6 oz)	448	7	14
burrito w/ beans & cheese	2 (6.5 oz)	377	7	12
burrito w/ beans & meat	2 (8.1 oz)	508	8	18
burrito w/ beef & chili peppers	2 (7.1 oz)	426	8	17
burrito w/ beef cheese & chili peppers	2 (10.7 oz)	634	10	25
chimichanga w/ beef & cheese	1 (6.4 oz)	443	11	23
enchilada w/ cheese & beef	1 (6.7 oz)	324	9	18
enchirito w/ cheese beef & beans	1 (6.8 oz)	344	8	16
frijoles w/ cheese	1 cup (5.9 oz)	226	4	8
nachos w/ cheese & jalapeno peppers	6 to 8 (7.2 oz)	607	14	34

FOOD	PORTION	CALS.	SAT. FAT	TOTAL FAT
nachos w/ cheese beans ground beef & peppers	6 to 8 (8.9 oz)	568	12	31
taco	1 sm (6 oz)	370	11	21
taco salad	1½ cups	279	7	15
taco shell baked	1 med (0.5 oz)	61	tr	3
tostada w/ beans & cheese	1 (5.1 oz)	223	5	10
tostada w/ guacamole	2 (9.2 oz)	360	10	23
Amy's Organic Enchilada Cheese	1 (4.7 oz)	210	3	9
Banquet Enchilada Chicken	1 pkg (11 oz)	360	3	10
Derby Tamales	2	160	3	7
Gebhardt Taco Shell	1	50	2	2
Healthy Choice Fiesta Chicken Fajitas	1 meal (7 oz)	260	1	4
Jimmy Dean Burrito Breakfast Bacon	1 (4 oz)	260	3	8
Life Choice Vegetable Enchilada Sonora	1 meal (14 oz)	420	0	2
Senor Felix's Empanadas Chicken	1 (4.7 oz)	340	30	15
Senor Felix's Tamales Blue Corn & Soy Cheese	2 + 4 tsp sauce (5.7 oz)	240	3	10
SPINACH				
fresh cooked	½ cup	21	tr	tr
frzn	½ cup	27	tr	tr
raw chopped	½ cup	6	tr	tr
spanakopita spinach pie	1 slice (3 x 4 in)	196	2	3
Stouffer's Creamed	½ cup (2.25 oz)	150	4	12
SPORTS BAR				
PowerBar Malt-Nut	1 bar (2.3 oz)	230	1	3
SPORTS DRINKS				
Gatorade Fruit Punch	1 cup (8 oz)	50	0	0
PowerAde Grape	8 fl oz	73	0	0
Slice All Sport Lemon Lime	8 fl oz	72	0	0
Snapple Sport Orange	1 bottle	80	0	0
SQUASH				
acorn cubed baked	½ cup	57	tr	tr
seeds salted & roasted	1 oz	148	2	12
spaghetti cooked	½ cup	23	tr	tr

FOOD	PORTION	CALS.	SAT. FAT	TOTAL FAT
SQUID				
fried	3 oz	149	2	6
STAR FRUIT				
fresh	1	42	0	tr
STRAWBERRIES				
fresh	1 cup	45	tr	1
Birds Eye Halved In Lite Syrup	½ cup	90	0	0
STUFFING/DRESSING				
bread	½ cup	195	2	8
STURGEON				
smoked	1 oz	48	tr	1
SUGAR				
maple	1 piece (1 oz)	100	0	tr
white	1 packet (6 g)	25	0	0
SUGAR SUBSTITUTES				
Equal Packet	1 pkg	4	0	0
NatraTaste Packet	1 pkg (1 g)	0	0	0
SugarTwin Packet	1 pkg (0.8 g)	3	0	0
Sweet One Packet	1 pkg (1 g)	4	0	0
Sweet'N Low Granulated	1 pkg (1g)	4	0	0
SUNFLOWER				
seeds roasted & salted	1 oz	165	1	14
SUSHI				
california roll	1 piece (0.8 oz)	28	tr	1
kim chi	⅓ cup (5.8 oz)	18	tr	tr
sashimi	1 serv (6 oz)	198	1	7
tuna roll	1 piece (0.7 oz)	23	tr	tr
vegetable roll	1 piece (1.2 oz)	27	tr	1
vinegared ginger	⅓ cup (1.6 oz)	48	tr	tr
wasabi	2 tsp (0.3 oz)	5	0	tr
yellowtail roll	1 piece (0.6 oz)	25	tr	1
SWEET POTATO				
baked w/ skin	1 (3.5 oz)	118	tr	tr
Royal Prince Candied	½ cup (4.9 oz)	210	0	1
SWISS CHARD				
fresh cooked	½ cup	18	0	tr

FOOD	PORTION	CALS.	SAT. FAT	TOTAL FAT
SWORDFISH				
cooked	3 oz	132	1	4
SYRUP				
maple	1 tbsp (0.8 oz)	52	0	0
Eden Barley Malt Organic Syrup	1 tbsp (0.7 fl oz)	60	0	0
Smucker's All Flavors Fruit Syrup	2 tbsp	100	0	0
TANGERINE				
fresh	1	37	tr	tr
Minute Maid Juice frzn	8 fl oz	120	0	0
TEA/HERBAL TEA				
brewed tea	6 oz	2	0	0
Bigelow Cinnamon Orange	5 fl oz	tr	—	tr
Bigelow Darjeeling Blend	5 fl oz	1	—	tr
Celestial Seasonings Lemon Zinger	8 fl oz	4	—	tr
Celestial Seasonings Naturally Decaffeinated	8 fl oz	10	—	1
Celestial Seasonings Sleepytime	8 fl oz	4	—	tr
Lipton Instant as prep	1 serv	0	0	0
Lipton Tea Bag Green Tea as prep	1	0	0	0
Lipton Tea Bag Quietly Chamomile as prep	1 cup	0	0	0
TEMPEH				
Lightlife Tempeh	½ cup	182	1	6
White Wave Burger	1 patty (3 oz)	110	0	3
TILEFISH				
cooked	3 oz	125	1	4
TOFU				
fresh fried	1 piece (0.5 oz)	35	tr	3
Mori-Nu Firm	1 in slice (3 oz)	50	0	3
Mori-Nu Lite Firm	1 in slice (3 oz)	35	0	1
Nasoya Silken	⅙ block (3 oz)	50	0	2
White Wave International Baked Oriental Teriyaki	¼ pkg (2 oz)	120	1	6
TOMATILLO				
fresh chopped	½ cup	21	—	1
TOMATO				
green	1	30	tr	tr

FOOD	PORTION	CALS.	SAT. FAT	TOTAL FAT
red	1 (4.5 oz)	26	tr	tr
sun dried	1 piece	5	tr	tr
sun dried in oil	1 piece (3 g)	6	tr	tr
Campbell Juice	6 oz	40	0	0
Contadina Italian Style Stewed	½ cup	40	0	0
Hebrew National Pickled	⅓ tomato (1 oz)	4	0	0
Mott's Clamato	8 fl oz	100	0	0
Ro-Tel Diced Tomatoes & Green Chilies	½ cup (4.4 oz)	20	0	0
Sonoma Pesto	¼ cup (2 oz)	110	2	9
Sonoma Tapenade	1 tbsp (0.7 oz)	70	1	6
TORTILLA				
Old El Paso Flour	1 (1.4 oz)	150	1	3
TROUT				
baked	3 oz	162	1	7
TUNA				
fresh cooked	3 oz	157	1	5
tuna salad	½ cup	159	1	8
tuna salad submarine sandwich w/ lettuce & oil	1	584	5	28
Bumble Bee Chunk Light In Oil	2 oz	160	3	12
Bumble Bee Chunk Light In Water	2 oz	60	1	1
TURBOT				
baked	3 oz	104	—	3
TURKEY				
breast	1 slice (0.75 oz)	23	tr	tr
breast w/ skin roasted	4 oz	212	2	8
dark meat w/ skin roasted	3.6 oz	230	4	12
Alpine Lace Breast Fat Free	2 oz	50	25	0
Empire Salami	3 slices (1.8 oz)	70	1	4
Healthy Choice Deli-Thin Roasted Breast	6 slices (2 oz)	60	1	2
Louis Rich Bologna	1 slice (1 oz)	50	1	4
Louis Rich Turkey Ham	4 slices (1.8 oz)	60	1	2
Perdue Breast Tenderloins Cooked	3 oz	110	1	1
Perdue Burger Cooked	1 (3 oz)	170	3	9

FOOD	PORTION	CALS.	SAT. FAT	TOTAL FAT
TURKEY SUBSTITUTES				
White Wave Meatless Sandwich Slices	2 slices (1.6 oz)	80	0	0
TURNIPS				
cooked mashed	½ cup (4.2 oz)	47	tr	tr
greens chopped cooked	½ cup	15	tr	tr
Southland Rutabaga Yellow Turnips frzn	4 oz	50	0	0
VEAL				
cutlet lean only fried	3 oz	156	1	4
ground broiled	3 oz	146	3	6
loin chop w/ bone lean & fat braised	1 chop (2.8 oz)	227	5	14
parmigiana	1 serv (4.2 oz)	279	10	18
VEGETABLE JUICE				
Muir Glen Organic	8 oz	70	0	0
V8 Original	6 fl oz	35	0	0
VEGETABLES MIXED				
caponata	¼ cup	28	—	1
curry	1 serv (7.7 oz)	398	—	33
pakoras	1 (2 oz)	108	—	5
peas & carrots	½ cup	48	tr	tr
ratatouille	½ cup	95	—	8
samosa	2 (4 oz)	519	—	46
Allen Okra Tomatoes & Corn	½ cup (4.1 oz)	30	0	0
Birds Eye Farm Fresh Broccoli And Cauliflower	¾ cup	30	0	0
Del Monte Mixed	½ cup (4.4 oz)	40	0	0
Hanover Vegetable Salad	½ cup	90	0	0
La Choy Chop Suey Vegetables	½ cup	10	tr	tr
Seneca Succotash	½ cup	90	0	0
VENISON				
roasted	3 oz	134	1	3
VINEGAR				
balsamic	1 tbsp	tr	0	0
WAFFLES				
plain	1 (7 in diam)	218	2	11
Belgian Chef Belgian	2 (2.5 oz)	140	1	3

FOOD	PORTION	CALS.	SAT. FAT	TOTAL FAT
Eggo Homestyle	2 (2.7 oz)	220	2	8
WALNUTS				
halves	1 oz	182	2	18
WATER				
Water Joe Caffeine Enhanced	8 fl oz	0	0	0
WATER CHESTNUTS				
Ka-Me Whole In Water	½ cup (4.5 oz)	45	0	0
WATERCRESS				
raw chopped	½ cup	2	tr	tr
WATERMELON				
fresh cut up	1 cup	50	—	1
fresh wedge	1/16	152	—	2
WAX BEANS				
Del Monte Cut Golden	½ cup (4.3 oz)	20	0	0
WHEAT				
Near East Taboule Salad	⅔ cup	120	1	3
White Wave Seitan	½ pkg (4 oz)	140	0	0
WHEAT GERM				
Kretschmer Original	¼ cup	103	1	3
WHIPPED TOPPINGS				
cream pressurized	1 tbsp	8	tr	tr
Kraft Whipped Topping	2 tbsp (0.4 oz)	20	1	2
Reddiwip Lite	2 tbsp (8 g)	15	0	1
WHITE BEANS				
dried cooked	1 cup	249	tr	1
Progresso Cannellini	½ cup (4.6 oz)	100	0	1
WHITEFISH				
smoked	1 oz	39	tr	tr
WILD RICE				
cooked	½ cup	83	tr	tr
WINE				
Boone's Delicious Apple	1 fl oz	21	0	0
Carlo Rossi Burgundy	1 fl oz	22	0	0
Carlo Rossi Chablis	1 fl oz	21	0	0
Carlo Rossi Red Sangria	1 fl oz	24	0	0
Fairbanks Cream Sherry	1 fl oz	42	0	0
Fairbanks Port	1 fl oz	44	0	0

FOOD	PORTION	CALS.	SAT. FAT	TOTAL FAT
Gallo Cabernet Sauvignon	1 fl oz	22	0	0
Gallo Chardonnay	1 fl oz	23	0	0
Gallo Zinfandel	1 fl oz	23	0	0
Sheffield Cellars Vermouth Extra Dry	1 fl oz	28	0	0
WINE COOLERS				
Bartles & Jaymes Original	12 fl oz	190	0	0
YAM				
S&W Candied	½ cup	180	0	0
YEAST				
brewer's	1 tbsp	25	tr	tr
YOGURT				
fruit lowfat snack size	4 oz	113	1	1
plain lowfat	8 oz	144	2	4
plain no fat	8 oz	127	tr	tr
Breyers Black Cherry Low Fat	8 oz	260	2	3
Breyers Red Raspberry Low Fat	8 oz	250	2	3
Cabot All Flavors	8 oz	220	2	3
Colombo Fat Free Banana Strawberry	8 oz	200	0	0
Colombo Fat Free Lemon	8 oz	170	0	0
Dannon Blended Nonfat Blueberry	6 oz	160	0	0
Dannon Blended Nonfat Peach	6 oz	150	0	0
Dannon Fruit On The Bottom Lowfat Mixed Berries	8 oz	240	2	3
Dannon Minipack Blended Nonfat Strawberry	4.4 oz	110	0	0
Dannon Sprinkl'ins Cherry Vanilla	4.1 oz	140	2	3
Dannon Tropifruta Nonfat Guava	6 oz	150	0	0
La Yogurt French Style Key Lime	6 oz	180	2	3
Light N'Lively Free Strawberry Fruit Cup	6 oz	170	0	0
Weight Watchers Cappuccino	1 cup	90	0	0
Weight Watchers Lemon	1 cup	90	0	0
Weight Watchers Strawberry	1 cup	90	0	0
YOGURT FROZEN				
Ben & Jerry's Cherry Garcia	½ cup (3.7 oz)	170	2	3
Ben & Jerry's No Fat Cappuccino	½ cup (3.3 oz)	140	0	0

FOOD	PORTION	CALS.	SAT. FAT	TOTAL FAT
Friendly's Fabulous Fudge Swirl	½ cup (2.6 oz)	140	3	3
Haagen-Dazs Chocolate	½ cup (3.4 oz)	160	2	3
Haagen-Dazs Fat Free Vanilla	½ cup (3.3 oz)	140	0	0
Tofutti Better Than Yogurt Chocolate Fudge	4 fl oz	120	1	2
Turkey Hill Nonfat Mint Cookie 'N Cream	½ cup (2.4 oz)	110	0	0
Turkey Hill Nonfat Vanilla Fudge	½ cup (2.4 oz)	110	0	0

ZUCCHINI

FOOD	PORTION	CALS.	SAT. FAT	TOTAL FAT
baby raw	1 (0.5 oz)	3	tr	tr
sliced cooked	½ cup	14	tr	tr
Del Monte With Italian Tomato Sauce	½ cup (4.2 oz)	30	0	0